KEEP RUNNING

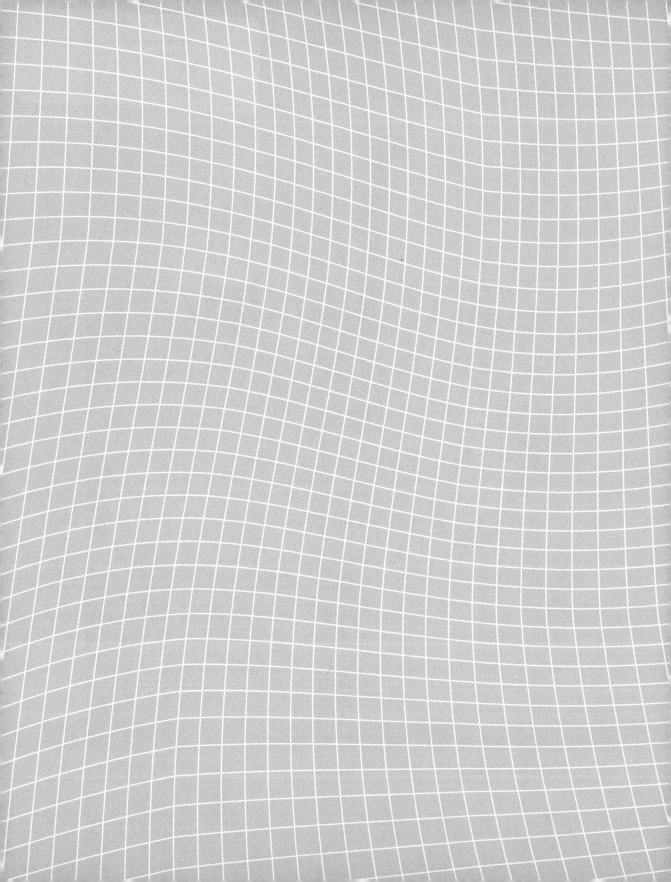

KEEP RUNNING

HOW TO RUN INJURY-FREE WITH POWER AND JOY FOR DECADES

Andrew Kastor

Illustrations by Rick Forgus

ROCKRIDGE
PRESS

Interior and Cover Designer: Brian Lewis
Art Producer: Megan Baggott
Editor: Rochelle Torke

Illustrations © 2020 Rick Forgus
Author photo by Miles Weaver

ISBN: Print 978-1-64611-444-3 | eBook 978-1-64611-445-0

R0

TO RUNNERS EVERYWHERE, MAY THE WIND FOREVER BE AT YOUR BACK

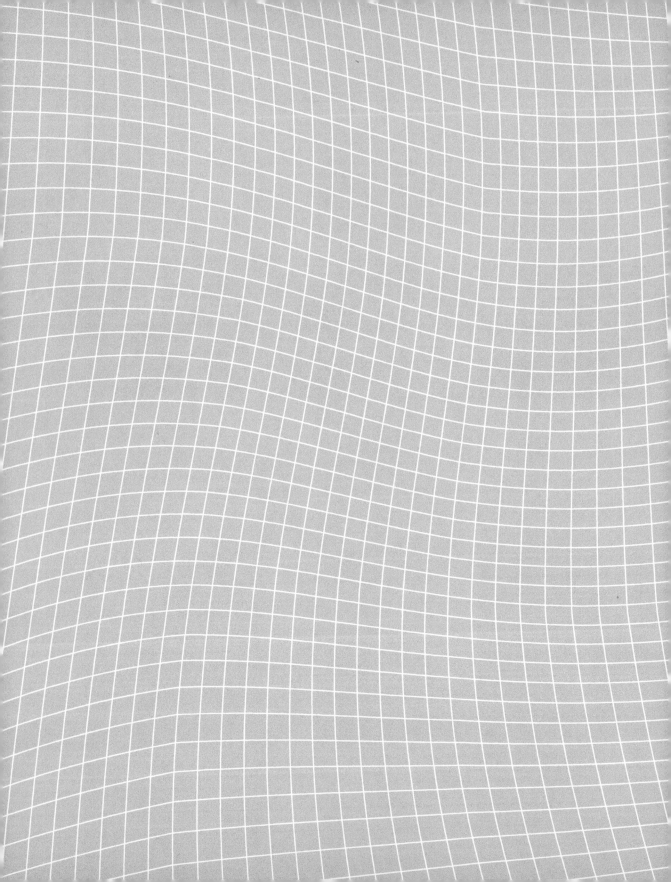

INTRODUCTION

Growing up in Southern California—where I was always near the beach and playing soccer—made it pretty easy to develop a love for running at a young age. But I didn't fully appreciate running as a sport in and of itself until my freshman year of high school, when I joined the cross-country team. I went into it as a way to get fit and gain speed for the upcoming winter soccer season, but I didn't know just how much I would fall for running. From the first race, I knew I'd found my true love. The early success I had in cross-country helped shape my confidence as a young teen, too. Transitioning to collegiate running only seemed natural, but I didn't even start on my team at Adams State University, a nationally ranked Division 2 school in Alamosa, Colorado. In fact, I was our seventh man in cross-country, while my roommates were all 4-minute milers.

I realized fairly quickly in college that running professionally was not in my cards, but the love affair I had with the sport only continued to grow. So I began to study physiology, human anatomy, kinesiology, and exercise science, grooming myself to potentially become a coach instead. I thrived in my studies—so much so that I started tutoring my teammates, the guys and ladies who were scoring all the points at our track meets.

After meeting my wife in 2000, we moved to Mammoth Lakes, California, about 300 miles north of where she and I grew up. It felt a little bit like moving back home, but with an added bonus of being by the mountains we'd come to love in Colorado. It was here, an ideal spot for training, that I started coaching a small group of runners (we only had six members our first year!) and created a club called the High Sierra Striders. Since then, I've been the coaching director for the Los Angeles Marathon and the head coach of the Mammoth Track Club, which has three divisions of athletes—elite (national and world-class), adults (5K to marathon), and youth.

Over the past 20 years, I've worked with runners of all ages and abilities, from fresh-out-of-college world-class athletes to middle-aged Boston Marathon qualifiers to 50-year-olds who are running their first 5Ks. One of the things I love most about this sport is that runners are an incredibly diverse group of people, from all different backgrounds and in all shapes and sizes. I enjoy every aspect of coaching different types of athletes. But I truly enjoy the dedicated ones the most, and these are often older individuals. These are men and women who enjoy being coached and are motivated by making progress. When athletes aren't dedicated, they fall off their training schedule and there's nothing I can do as a coach to get them back on track. My goal is to get my athletes to a place where they are self-driven and just need a little guidance, so I can use my knowledge to point them in the right direction. I'm not a hand-holder, but I'll give a gentle nudge toward the right path. These are the runners who really take off, and it is a joy to be a part of their journey.

This sport has been so good to my wife and me that we are always looking for ways to give back to the running community. We want to support up-and-coming Olympians. We want to give the youth in our area a chance to experience track and field, and we want to give local adults an opportunity to be a part of a team that can lift them up both on and off the track every week.

By simply picking up and reading this book, I believe you are passionate about our sport, too. Whether you're chasing personal records in multiple distances or simply cruising around your neighborhood every now and then, I want you to keep running strong throughout your life, well into your 70s, 80s, and beyond. It's possible, I promise. There are many runners who have forged this path before us.

I know you have concerns about how your body will hold up over time. I know you're thinking that your fastest times are behind you. I know you may feel like younger people at races or down at the local track might look at you funny or think that you shouldn't be running so hard. These are all valid concerns, and I hear you. But it doesn't have to be this way . . . and it doesn't mean you should stop running.

I am 42 years old. I used to be fast in college. I know that I will never run a 4:12 mile again; heck, even 5:12 would be challenging. Over the past few years, my goals and priorities have shifted to this basic principle: "Just get in the miles, get out the door, put one foot in front of the other, and do it."

As a coach who works with elite athletes, I need to always have the mind-set of optimizing every aspect of our lives to perform our best. From sleep, to diet, to recovery, to training workouts, we're always trying to find ways to gain an edge over the competition. You are no different. The goal is simply to run farther rather than faster. And if you optimize your training and your lifestyle, you too can run joyfully and injury-free for years to come.

Our thoughts control our actions; therefore, we must maintain a healthy mind-set when continuing to run and train (and live!) as we age. We need to work on being kind to ourselves, accepting and flexible enough to roll with the changes in our mind and body. Having a more positive thought process will help you adapt in the years to come, eventually allowing you to totally reinvent yourself as a master or senior runner.

There are some master runners out there who are absolutely crushing their competition. Sixty-year-old men running under-3-hour marathons, 50-year-old women running 19-minute 5Ks. These outliers either reinvented themselves as master athletes or they were once great collegiate runners, now finding ways to continue along their path of high-level training and racing as they get older. Either way, you can be just like them. We're all genetically different, sure, but we can still make the same lifestyle choices and goals to get us there. Your success ultimately depends on how badly you want it. How hard are you willing to work and how much time are you able to dedicate to pursue your goals?

Listening to your body and paying attention to how it reacts to certain types of training stimulus will be your greatest asset in running strong into your golden years. Check in with yourself regularly, be smart, and plan accordingly. Use the wisdom you've acquired from years of living and training to guide you, lean into your support crew, keep your head up, and remember: All you really need to do is put one foot in front of the other.

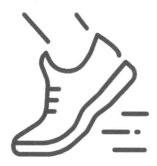

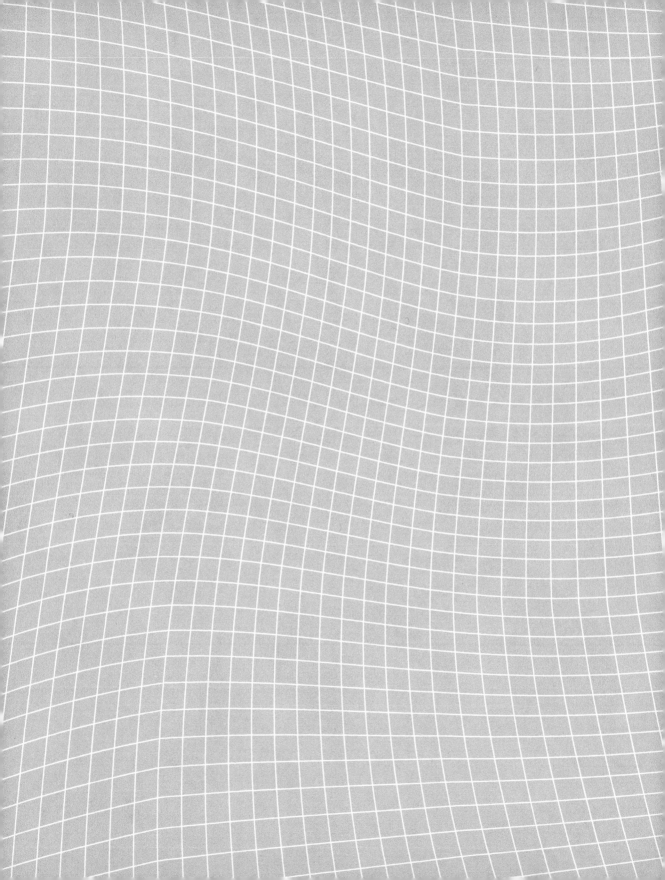

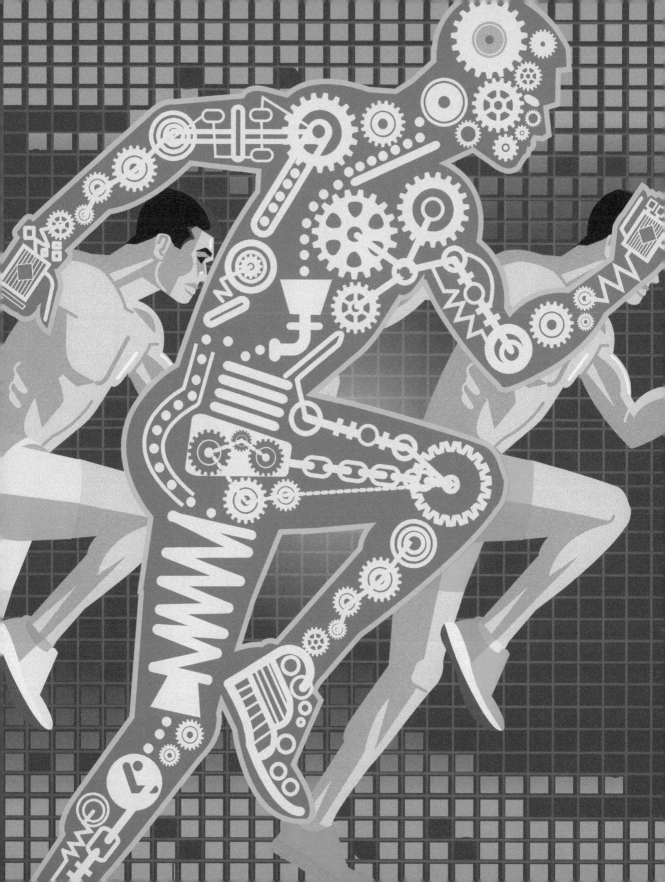

CHAPTER ONE

INSPIRATION

THE HUMAN RUNNING MACHINE

We are built to run. Everything about the physical makeup of human beings indicates that we were designed for long-distance running. Through evolution, we made the leap from the trees to the ground to hunt for food or track down other animals. Early humans evolved into great distance runners by developing specific traits, such as long tendons and ligaments in their feet (to act as springs) and shoulders that rotated independently of their heads (to counteract the rotational torque of their hips) that would help get them from point A to point B faster.

In addition to all of the structural adaptations human evolution gave us as runners, our bodies also create hormones that allow us to run for longer periods of time, numbing the pain and discomfort that our feet, ankles, and knees endure. These hormones are called endorphins, otherwise known as the chemical that gives us the famous "runner's high." This "high" stems from the days when we were hunting on the plains and chasing down our prey, sometimes for hours at a time.

Over the course of this book, we'll explore the how's and why's of running and the role aging plays in it. We'll take a deep dive into what you can expect from your running, racing, and lifestyle down the road. We'll get deep in the weeds on how to navigate each decade—how to train, what to eat, when to eat, what lifestyle changes you'll want to consider, and how to have a positive outlook on the aging process.

YOU'RE NEVER TOO OLD

Hear me out: You're never too old to run. If anyone ever tells you that, it's a myth. Age alone does not decide anything—other than whether we get to vote, drink at bars, or get discounts at the movie theater, that is. So let's go ahead and get this all cleared up and bust some of the other most common myths on aging:

 MYTH: You shouldn't engage in intense exercise as you get older.

A popular thought is that the older we get, the higher the probability is that we'll get hurt, so we should limit the amount of high-intensity exercise we perform. But there is no research to back this up, so listen to your body and do what feels good for you (with your doctor's approval, of course!).

 MYTH: Due to hormonal shifts as we age, we tend to get fatter.

Negative! While it is widely known that our hormones do shift and their productivity declines with age, gaining weight only happens when we have a poor diet, overeat, and stop exercising.

 MYTH: Running is more painful as you get older.

Experiencing the common aches and pains associated with running does not mean that our bodies are wearing out. By taking good care of yourself, eating well, sleeping well, and focusing on recovery, our knees and other body parts should work properly and pain-free for decades. There's no reason that running should be painful at any age.

 MYTH: Running ages you faster.

Umm, no! The perception that getting too thin or losing the fat surrounding your face will give you that old gaunt look is B.S. But getting wrinkles or doing anything outside without sunscreen will certainly age anyone.

 MYTH: Running uses up your heartbeat quota.

Some believe we're born with a fixed allotment of heartbeats for our lifetime, and we can use them up faster by running. This idea is superstitious at best. Very simply, running makes your heart stronger and regular exercise is recommended by the American Heart Association to live longer.

SEASONED RUNNING HEROES

If you've been running for a few decades and occasionally read *Runner's World* magazine or the now out-of-print *Running Times*, chances are you know about Ed Whitlock, the Canadian master-class running and racing phenom who passed away in 2017. In 2003, Whitlock set a world masters record for breaking three hours in the marathon as someone over the age of 70. At 73, he ran the Toronto Waterfront Marathon in a ridiculously impressive 2:54.49. Ed had three running careers during his time on this planet—he was a 4:31 miler in high school; a world masters champion in the 800m and 1500m in his 40s; and then a superhero of sorts in his 60s, rewriting all the senior world records, from the 5K to the marathon.

During his late 60s and early 70s, Ed would routinely perform a few three-hour runs per week, along with his other workouts. It didn't matter if he just plodded along at a pace that was slightly quicker than a crawl—he was spending time on his feet, up to 100 miles per week! His idea of training was to log as many miles as he possibly could, no matter what the pace, which was usually somewhere between an 8- to 11-minute mile. What's interesting about this is that he actually ran all of his races between a 5:45- to 7-minute mile pace. For fun, he would routinely run through a cemetery during training, saying that it reminded him of his own mortality.

Another inspirational runner in her 60s is the incomparable Joan Benoit Samuelson. I've had the great pleasure of getting to know Joan over the years. She was the first Olympic gold medalist in the women's marathon in 1984. Today, she still continues to tear up the road-racing scene; in 2019, at 62, she ran the Berlin Marathon in 3:02.

Joan maintains a simple lifestyle nowadays, frequently traveling around the world to promote races and organizations. She has personally won many of the races she visits, such as the Boston and Chicago Marathons. It's obvious that Joan has a competitive spirit that has driven her to not only push her body in training all these years, but also to allow for proper recovery so she could continue to run strong.

I've been coaching my friend Sherryl Taylor, who is now an avid runner in her 70s, on and off for about 15 years now. She and her husband, Tony, live in Mammoth Lakes, have been married for 50-plus years and have a lovely family with kids and grandkids.

Sherryl wasn't too competitive in her earlier years. Instead, she was busy raising a family, pursuing her volunteer work, and traveling. It really wasn't until her late 50s that she started to train harder, running intervals on the track (that she helped the Mammoth Track Club build and fund-raise for in 2012!), performing hill repeats, tempo runs, and marathon simulation runs. One of her best performances came at the 2005 Chicago Marathon, where she placed third in her age group (60–64). Since then, she has maintained a steady diet of two to three half-marathons per year.

AGE IS REALLY A STATE OF MIND

It's often the ones who start running late in life who I love to coach the most. It's inspiring to guide them through the process of training and plotting a yearly calendar of races. It's all so new and they're driven to do a good job, to be the best they can be in a new sport they're confident they can master. Also, the ones that start later in life have had fewer injuries and less scar tissue to deal with. The newbies can see progress right away, and that's always exciting for both the athlete and their coach.

A common thread among the athletes that I've mentioned is that they all have a great attitude toward aging. They have successfully adapted to getting older and are excited to reinvent themselves through an activity that only about 15 percent of the US population participates in each year.

Maintaining a positive attitude becomes increasingly important as that clock continues to tick. Saying "I can" or "I will" when met with a challenge becomes increasingly difficult. It takes courage, motivation, and vitality to keep pursing your goals and dreams.

During the course of this book, we will identify key habits and mind-sets of folks of all ages who have pursued running with renewed vigor. I'll share tips that will help provide the support you need to run powerfully and energetically well into your 70s, 80s, and 90s.

The world's population is aging rapidly. According to the World Health Organization (WHO), the number of people aged 60 or older will rise from 900 million to 2 billion between 2015 and 2050 (from 12 to 22 percent of the global population). WHO states that "there's no 'typical' older person." They've found that some 80-year-olds have physical and mental capacities similar to many 20-year-olds. They also state that good physical and mental health in older people is not random but is directly influenced by their physical and social environments. Good habits for healthy living generally start during young adulthood and having access to health care plays a large role later in life.

THE GOLDEN YEARS AS A RUNNER

Despite what you might think, growing old does have some perks, hence why they're called the "golden years." You've become better at everything you've learned throughout your lifetime. This is called "crystallized intelligence," or the accumulation of knowledge and facts that you're then able to apply to certain situations, helping further your progress in those areas.

Over the years, I've had running clients tell me they were nervous about a certain race or event or that they felt like they were behind in their training and preparation, which ultimately led to less confidence. I'd try to reassure them by saying, "Okay, you may not have had the best buildup for this marathon, but you've done this time and time again for years, sometimes decades. You have the experience required to toe that line and get the job done, no matter what." That way, when they cross the finish line, they're usually very proud of their performance, even if it's not a personal best or they missed earning a spot on the podium.

We all know that age is just a number. You can either be a young 50 or an old 50—it's your choice. You can also be an old 30, really. Good genes play a factor in whether or not you'll be breaking masters running records, but being fit and fast at 50 or 60 years old . . . well, that's totally up to you. The knowledge of how to feel your best and train strong as you get older is out there; you just have to seek it out. You're reading this book, so I know you're already on the right path. Good job!

TAKING AGEISM IN STRIDE

Our culture tends to be incredibly youth-centric. The world of sports is no exception to the rule. There are so many sports clubs and organizations for developing young athletes, and parents pour billions of dollars each year into the development of their children's skills, hoping they'll someday receive a sports scholarship and become the next great Olympian.

At the same time, the US lacks a goc port structure of sports and fitness aging population. But each year, it is getting better and better, with senior leagues popping up around the country.

In the past, older Americans were frequently portrayed as lonely or in dire need of care. But this perception is incredibly outdated. There are 110 million people aged 50 and older in this country, and according to AARP, "it's definitely time for the creative industries to update their mind-set about the 50-plus demographic." In 2019, AARP released a stereotype-shattering collection of images and videos showing people in their 50s enjoying fitness and a variety of other fun, healthy activities. These types of campaigns are essential in order to erase the notion that "old" has to mean slow and frail.

WHO has stated that experiencing ageism can reduce an older person's social interactions, harm their health, and reduce their lifespan. Those with their own negative attitudes about aging tend to recover more slowly when injured or disabled. I repeat: Having a good mind-set as you get older is so, so important.

I personally believe we're involved in a sport that is very welcoming to all ages and walks of life. In our little mountain town of 7,000 people, we have a widely diverse track club—it includes recent college graduates, attorneys, working professionals, retirees, first-timers, seasoned veterans, and elite athletes. Running is the tie that binds us, making us almost like one big (sweaty) family.

In theory, the longer you live, the more experiences you have and the wiser you become. If you recognize ageism both internally and externally, just know that you have the ability to combat its negative effects. Say to yourself, "I deserve to run as hard as I like. I deserve to run the races I choose to. No one knows whether it's a good or bad idea better than I do."

In the context of this book, I'm a bit on the younger side, at 42 years old, and I haven't experienced much in terms of ageism, yet. But I plan to practice what I preach going into my senior years and applaud all runners older than me who are training out there.

DIVERSITY IN RUNNING

Is ageism the new sexism? Kathrine Switzer broke the glass ceiling for women by running the Boston Marathon in 1967—she was the first female finisher of the event. Believe it or not, at the time people honestly thought that women were not physically built for running, that somehow their female parts would fall out if they ran more than a few miles at a time. Switzer trained like everyone else and knew she could compete in Beantown, but she

was met with one major obstacle during the race: the event director. He physically tried to stop her from running, but Switzer's boyfriend wouldn't have it, so he body slammed the director to the ground. She ran for equality. Now Kathrine claims that "we are into the next revolution, which is aging."

With the number of baby boomers (or just "boomers" as they're being called now) on the rise, I think Kathrine is onto something. Unfortunately, she feels like she—and other women—are experiencing the same prejudice they did 50 years ago; then for being a woman, now for being older. The prejudice stems from claims that older people are too weak or too fragile and that they should slow down.

Switzer recognizes this perception is slowly starting to shift for the better, now that more seniors are completing marathons and half-marathons. She feels like there's an opportunity to show millennials how to live a long and healthy lifestyle, leading by example.

RUNNING: AN EVOLUTIONARY LOVE STORY

From an evolutionary standpoint, we are born to run long distances. Millions of years ago, we appeared as hunters and gatherers. Usually in small packs, we would chase down our prey. Most of the animals on the savannah possessed more fast-twitch muscle fibers than us, and were therefore much better at running short distances, but they also produced a tremendous amount of heat and needed to take frequent breaks in the shade.

THE ANCIENT HUMAN HISTORY OF RUNNING

Early humans were just fast enough and had plenty of endurance to keep animals in a galloping-type gait, which left them unable to pant and expel heat. As long as the pack of hunters jogged ahead at a steady clip, they could keep their prey in a galloping mode behind them, forcing them into heat exhaustion after 15 to 20 minutes. We can still outrun nearly all mammals on the planet after about 15 minutes, especially on a really hot day, due to our hairless bodies and enlarged sweat glands.

Whether you like the concept of chasing down your own meals or not (hello, vegetarians!), we can all agree that running made us human. One hypothesis stated that, thanks to our ability to successfully chase down mammals for food and get plenty of protein in our meals, our brains were able to develop and evolve into what they are today. Aerobic exercise also causes the anterior hippocampus (the area of our brains involved with memory) and several other regions of our brains to grow in size,

not to mention the fact that exercise makes us stronger and healthier in general.

Bipedalism (our ability to run on two feet) is how we were eventually able to carry sharp weapons to use on our prey once they succumbed to heat exhaustion. The tired animal would have no chance of escape when a pack of *Homo sapiens* tracked it to its final resting spot. Our ancestors also developed fine tracking skills (no GPS needed!) with their larger brains. They'd look for animal tracks in the dirt or broken blades of grass left by their prey. Remember, humans had to compete against other carnivores, like lions and hyenas on the savannah, so we had to be fast, strong, and smart to survive.

Through evolution and our desire to grow as a dominant species, *Homo sapiens* (and earlier versions of humans) sought out protein to boost both fitness and intelligence. Along with becoming smarter as a result, they also became more anatomically efficient so they could chase down their prey.

Here's a list of many of the optimal skeletal adaptations that were made from head to toe:

1. A balanced head (to be more stabilized while in pursuit of our prey)

2. A tall, narrow body (to maintain a lower body temperature)

3. Narrow hips (for better counter-rotation of our torsos)

4. Longer legs than arms (for improved stride length)

5. Long Achilles tendon and an arch in the foot (to preserve energy when running)

6. Strong position of the big toe (for better toe-off)

7. Shorter "little" toes (for added stability)

Through crystallized intelligence, the older, wiser ancient people traveled with their hunting groups, sharing their knowledge and experience with the younger, faster hunters.

There's also evidence that older runners in a village would run long distances to visit other remote villages. They spoke several native dialects and could share successful agricultural techniques and other useful topics for survival and growth.

RUNNING AS A MODERN COMPETITION

Later on in history, the Greeks used runners to deliver messages from village to village. Most famously, Pheidippides delivered the news from Marathon to Athens (a 25-mile trip) that the Greeks had defeated the Persian Army, but also warned that they might launch another attack in Athens. The legend goes that Pheidippides was so exhausted after running the first-ever recorded "marathon" in about three hours that he died right there on the spot.

Athens hosted the first modern-day Olympics in 1896. During the Games, people from around the world kept up with the results via newspaper and telegraph. The Boston Athletic Association (BAA) got word that a very long-distance run (24 miles) had been contested. They thought, "Why don't we just host one of these races in Boston?" Thus giving birth to the world's oldest—and most prestigious—contested marathon.

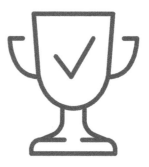

The US had several running booms starting in the 1970s. Road running in the 1960s truly seemed to be the bastard child of track and field, and marathons were few and far between—even the Boston Marathon only had about 1,000 participants at the time. By the 1970s, running had creative energy behind it and sponsors offered prize money to elite athletes. In other words, it had become commercialized for the betterment of the sport. Running shoes were becoming a thing, and it was estimated that 25 million Americans took up some aspect of running, or jogging, as it was more often referred to back then.

No book about running would be complete without mentioning the great US Olympic Marathon Champion (1972) Frank Shorter. He's heavily credited with the running boom of the 1970s. The television coverage of the Games in Munich that summer changed running forever. Folks in the US watched as Frank ran his last lap with a German imposter in front of him who had entered the stadium just moments before. The ABC commentator, Jim McKay, turned this spectacle into a dramatic event in Olympic history and (finally!) placed the sport of marathoning in the cultural spotlight.

WHAT THE WORLD'S GREATEST RUNNERS TEACH US

We can learn a lot from the world's greatest runners, including aging Olympic athletes and runners who are competing at the World Master Track and Field Championships or World Senior Games. These individuals inspire and motivate us, while also teaching us how to remain competitive among those in our age group.

I follow many running clubs and organizations on social media, so when I scroll through my Instagram and Twitter feeds, I occasionally come across videos like "100-year-old man breaks world record!" It's usually a video of a 100m track race, during which there are only six or seven competitors racing for the national 90-plus age group championship. It's the greatest thing! So inspiring. Yes, there are a lot of negative things out there on social media. Trust me, I know. That's why I choose to focus my attention on the positive posts, pictures, and videos. We need more exposure for runners in their 70s, 80s, and beyond competing and breaking records. These clips will hopefully help defy some of the negative stereotypes about older athletes and inspire others to get out there, too.

When I come across these videos, I inevitably ask myself, "Will I be able to run like that when I'm that age? What will it take to get there?" I know I'll have to sleep and eat well every single day from here on out in order to make it to a starting line at 100 years old, but I'm up for it.

How are these centenarians doing it? Is it just good genetics?

> "WHEN WE GET OLDER, IT IS EASIER AND EASIER TO BLAME OUR RELATIVES FOR OUR OWN HEALTH PROBLEMS. WE GET DIAGNOSED WITH HIGH CHOLESTEROL, AND IT'S BECAUSE OUR DAD AND UNCLE DIED DUE TO HEART DISEASE. IF WE PUT OUR CELL PHONE IN THE MICROWAVE, IT'S BECAUSE GRANDMA HAD A SLIGHT CASE OF DEMENTIA. BUT THIS ISN'T HOW GENES WORK."
>
> — From the book, *You: Staying Young* by Michael F. Roizen, M.D. and Mehmet C. Oz, M.D.

Your genetic destiny is not inevitable. If you're unhappy with the genes you've been given, you can protect yourselves from genetic abnormalities. Your longevity and success as an athlete are based 25 percent on your genetics and 75 percent on your behavior and lifestyle choices. Identical twin studies should convince you that how we choose to live—our behavioral choices—make up a majority of how healthy we are. Compound that over decades of living and it can really add up!

My wife, Deena, is adopted. When she goes to the doctor's office and has to fill out the patient intake forms, it goes something like this. She reads: "Please indicate any major conditions/illnesses that your immediate family members have had below." And then she simply writes, "N/A."

Deena goes through life doing the best she can without knowing if her biological mother has/had diabetes or if her biological grandmother had dementia (or thyroid issues, cancer, or fill in the blank). So as a precautionary measure (and because she's an amazing person and an elite runner), she eats well, exercises, gets adequate sleep and recovery, reads and writes, uses painting as a creative outlet, and keeps herself intellectually stimulated to ward off the possibility of developing memory loss. She's leading a healthy, balanced lifestyle.

RUNNING TRADITIONS AROUND THE WORLD

Some running experts would argue that Japan is the most running-obsessed culture in the world. Running is the number two sport there, just behind baseball. At the elite level, the Japanese hold annual relay races called Ekiden, and major corporations and universities send their best teams to compete. Very few of the elite Japanese distance runners compete outside of Japan. These runners care more about competing for their teams than traveling for world events, unless it's the Tokyo Marathon, of course. Unfortunately, it's all too common for coaches to overtrain their athletes and persistently run them on concrete, asphalt, and other hard surfaces.

In East Africa, on the other hand, they pride themselves on running on soft surfaces and competing (very well!) globally. Some of the best runners in this part of the world attend American universities and high schools, competing against American kids for scholarships.

In marathon running, it's often the African nations versus everyone else. The countries of Kenya, Ethiopia, Eritrea, Uganda, Algeria, and Morocco dominate the global running scene. Why? In most of these countries, running is the number one sport and provides a chance for people to earn a living—at least for a few years of competing on the road-running circuit. I personally think that the US and Europe have the same amount of genetic talent as the African nations. We just offer a wider variety of sports for our youth to participate in, which dilutes the running pool a bit. This is not a complaint, mind you—freedom of choice is way more important—it's just an observation.

We can learn a lot about ourselves from these running-centric cultures. If running was the only sport we participated in and the pride of our country was on the line every time we competed, then we'd probably be faster, too. When our mind, body, and spirit are all on the same page—putting one foot in front of the other for miles and miles, day after day, week after week, year after year, our bodies become increasingly efficient at running, just through repetition. When training for a marathon, the more you train at race pace, the easier it will get and the more likely you'll be able to complete 26.2 miles at a steady clip.

Side note: The US has been slowly rising in competition on the global stage. We've brought many medals home from both the World Track and Field Championships and the Olympic Games since 2016.

THE RARÁMURI TRIBE

In 2011, Christopher McDougall wrote a groundbreaking book called *Born to Run*, about the Tarahumara Indian tribe from the Copper Canyons of Arizona. Also called Rarámuri (or "runners on foot"), this tribe is composed of indigenous people living in the state of Chihuahua, Mexico. They are known for their remarkable running endurance and their ability to log countless miles wearing sandals fashioned from old tires found in the desert. This community makes its home in the cliffs and leads a fairly simple lifestyle.

It's not uncommon for the Rarámuri to cover up to 200 miles in one run, over hills, rocks, and vegetation. They do it with such joy in their hearts, too. Maybe that's their secret? They have a storied history of performing 100-mile-plus races dating as far back as the 1860s, when they competed against neighboring villages for fun.

Maybe it's the simplicity of their running that allows them to go for hours on end. You'll find no GPS watches charging in their homes. They don't know the paces they're running and wouldn't care if you told them. They just run from point A to point B as fast as they can. And based on the distance, they also calibrate their sustained effort to precisely allocate their energy expenditure.

When the Tarahumara run and take breaks, they drink water, eat snacks, and sit down immediately (preferably in the shade)—no standing around and wasting precious energy. They have a particular focus on efficiency, with life and with running. Along these lines, when they run, their pace and effort is steady, and their heart rate remains the same, whether they're going uphill or down.

Additionally, they work as a team, running together during training and racing. No one is out there running by themselves—it's always done as a pack, and they feed off each other's energy. It's apparent that the Tarahumara run and race with joy. They run with a spiritual significance, which spurs them on to do great things and allows them to better endure the pain and discomfort normally felt in the later stages of a 200-mile run or ultra-marathon.

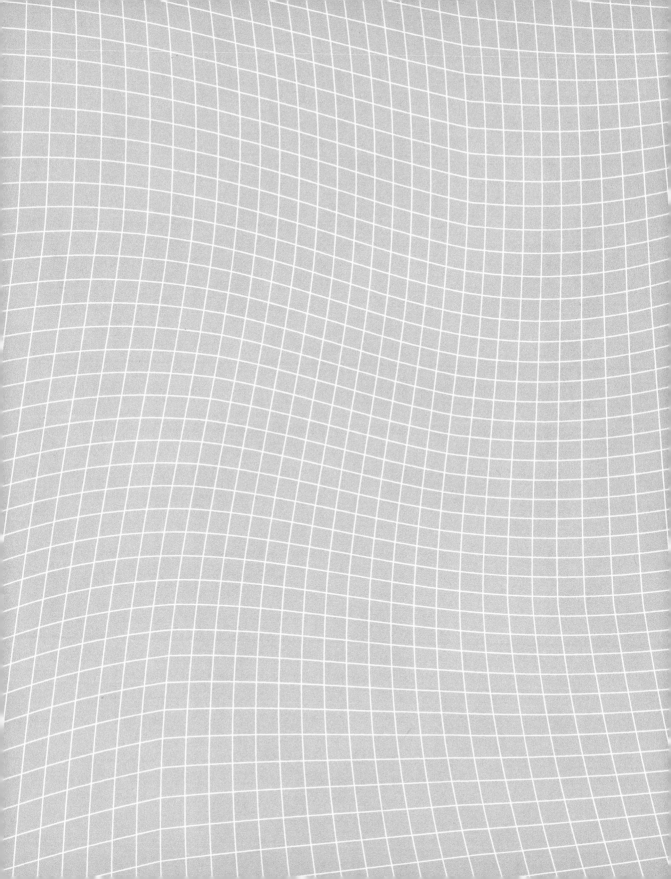

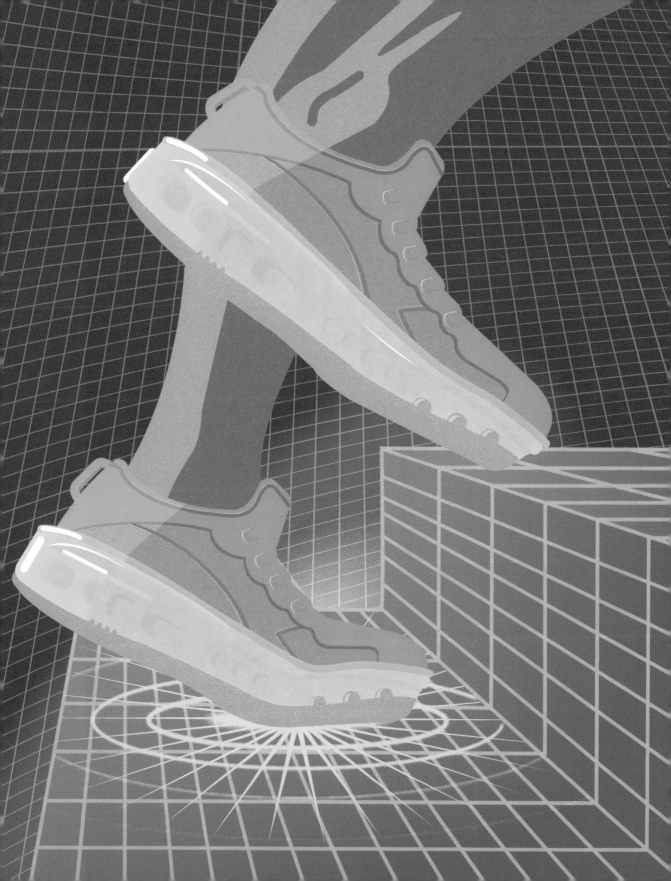

CHAPTER TWO

OPTIMIZATION

REFINING YOUR APPROACH BY DECADE

We are slowing down a little; that's okay, it's natural. The good news is that we're still going, and moving forward at any speed is much better than the alternative, right? (Research shows that runners who stick with regular training and racing routines slow down a little—about 0.5 to 1 percent—every year throughout their 40s, 50s, and 60s.) Whether you were a competitive athlete in high school or college, like me, or you've always been chasing your own personal records as a recreational runner, the process of aging, combined with work, family, and other life obligations, may mean your fastest race times are behind you.

One thing I've found that keeps running enjoyable over the years is training with others, especially those with like-minded goals and similar ages. Where I live, in Mammoth Lakes, California, my wife, Deena, and I lead a running organization called the Mammoth Track Club, which comprises runners of all ages and abilities. We have elite athletes, like Deena, who is a three-time Olympian, Olympic Bronze Medalist, and the American record holder in the marathon (2 hours, 19 minutes and 36 seconds); adult recreational runners, many of whom have never run on a track before; age group racers; and young athletes. We host a track practice every Tuesday from April to October. Every now and then, I survey our adult members and ask them what they're training for, why they enjoy the club atmosphere, and whether or not they would run repeat intervals on their own. Every single time, the answer to the latter is a resounding no. As we age, the two main factors that contribute to our running decline are drops in our VO_2 Max (your maximal oxygen uptake) and our muscles' ability to produce power.

TIPS BY DECADE

AGE GROUP	COMPETITIVE CONSIDERATIONS	TRAINING FOCUS
35–44	Consider yourself a young master's runner. You might be coming off some personal records in the 10K, half-marathon and/or marathon distance and you're kind of secretly looking forward to joining the 40-year-old age group so you can be one of the faster ones (maybe for a change). Longer distances are still approachable and hitting new PRs in the half-marathon or marathon is totally achievable. Life is very busy, so finding balance is necessary. You are fierce, competitive, and have a killer instinct.	Your training shouldn't look too different from when you were in your 20s and early 30s, but rest and sleep become increasingly more important. It might be time to consider adding one more recovery day in between your hard training sessions and long runs. Or maybe it's time to add an aerobic cross-training workout into your weekly routine—you can use it as a recovery workout or just something to get your heart rate up and make you sweat a little more than usual. And be sure to incorporate some hill repeats into your routine.
45–54	Look forward to being the youngest—and/ or fittest—competitor in your age group! You have a chance to really clean up, bringing home age-group medals and awards! You're just going to need to start incorporating things into your routine that help keep you fit and healthy, like consistent weight training, and longer running warm-up and cool-down sessions.	With your ability to recover gradually decreasing each year, you might want to consider switching your current 7-day training cycle to a 10-day training cycle. You'll take 1 to 2 days off and cross-train 1 to 2 days every cycle. Since we lose a bit of power each year as well, it would be wise to lengthen the recovery intervals in your workouts by 25 to 50%.

REST AND RECOVERY

You've probably got a lot going on in life with work, family, and friends. Your body might be willing to press hard 2 to 3 times per week, but you need to ask yourself if adequate sleep is there, too. Ideally, you'll go to a massage therapy session every couple weeks, and if nothing else, do foam rolling and self-massages as much as possible. If you're going to crank up your training in an attempt to be more competitive, then you need to make sure there is ample recovery happening outside of running to reap the rewards.

If possible, take a nap after your long run each week. Schedule those massage therapy appointments in advance. Give yourself plenty of time in the mornings to eat a nutritious breakfast, hydrate well, and, of course, get your workouts in before work. Start relying on your experience during training and racing and make sure you listen to your body's little aches and pains.

MIND-SET

Personal bests are still possible, particularly in the longer-distance events that require more endurance and experience. Experience, yes, you've got it! You can be more relaxed going into races now, too. You've been there and done that, you know the drill. Also, now that you're a more responsible adult, if you can, treat yourself to nicer accommodations—and healthier meals—on race weekends, travel a day earlier, schedule a massage every 2 to 4 weeks during training, and spend time taking care of your body. Be competitive with people in your age group and the one below.

Don't get upset with your training and racing times. Start referring to age-graded performance charts (you can find them online) to keep your motivation up. This is a great way for you to more accurately compare your stats to those of the younger runners who are breaking the tape every race. Be confident in your abilities and rely on your race experience to guide you to consistent performances throughout the year.

TIPS BY DECADE

AGE GROUP	COMPETITIVE CONSIDERATIONS	TRAINING FOCUS
55–64	The great news is there are less competitors in your age group now! So you're basically guaranteed some sort of racing win in your near future. At this age, and from here on out, simply show up to the starting line healthy and undertrained—easy!	Theme: undertrain. Show up to each workout healthy, feeling good, and well prepared, then just follow your instincts; the ones you've been developing for decades as a runner. Warm-ups are critical, so be sure you start your workouts walking, then break into a jog to ease into the pace. Keep those hill repeats in your plan as well—one session every 7 to 14 days should do the trick.
65–74	Show up, get the work in, and go home. You don't need to prove yourself to anyone else or do anything fancy on the track. Get to the starting line healthy and you'll win, in addition to inspiring other younger competitors.	Hang around younger runners at the local track. Don't listen to anyone who brings you down and says that you shouldn't be running hard or competing at your age. They're just jealous that you're out there crushing 10Ks each month. Disclaimer: Listen to your doctor's advice; he or she may tell you to curb your intensity for a reason. Use races as your speed work. Keep the hill repeats in your training plan—once every day can help keep your power up.
75+	Congrats! Most races, you'll be one of the few in your age group. That alone is worth celebrating. Be sure to have on shoes that are comfortable and functional (and have less than 300 miles on them). Get a new uniform, too, and be sure to get your name printed on it so folks can cheer for you during the race and at practice. You're pretty much the closest thing to a celebrity they might see today.	You're going to start drastically reducing your running volume and training time. Go to the alternating On Day, Off Day approach. And dedicate one day per week to working on turnover by doing some easy strides on a track or field. Let the races be your threshold work and race sparingly to allow for recovery.

REST AND RECOVERY

I have one more piece of advice for you: TAKE NAPS. Lots and lots of naps. Getting that extra shot of human growth hormone (HGH) while you sleep is critical for your recovery after a hard training session. By now, you should be working out every 3 to 4 days and cross-training 2 days per week to alleviate acute and chronic inflammation.

Not much is different from the last decade, but you need to be better about listening to your body. By now you should have settled into a cross-training routine that you're comfortable with. Sleep will, of course, be dependent on how hard you're training now. If you're only doing one workout per week, then the demand for sleep might not be as great.

Most runs should now be considered "recovery runs." There is not a huge need for dedicated speed workouts. Just getting out the door on healthy legs is your goal. Start each run with a short walk to limber you up. Get in some strides to maintain power and dynamic flexibility.

MIND-SET

It's okay (ideal, really) to start off each and every run with a walk to warm up your joints. When it's cold out, be sure to wear extra layers that you can easily shed throughout your run. Ask yourself, "Do I still enjoy this? Am I making progress and getting satisfaction from putting in the miles?" If the answers are all yes, then keep at it. If not, you might want to consider shifting your focus. Find comfort in your training log, your race bib numbers, and the medals that you've accumulated over the years.

Just keep turning your legs over. Accept that you are now an inspiration on the track, an icon. Men and women in their 20s and 30s will aspire to be you, even if you think you're running pretty darn slow. There should be more time in your schedule for recovery, exploring new trails, meeting new people, and traveling to dreamy destination races.

You are an inspiration. Running is not only a way to improve yourself and your personal journey, but it's also a way to inspire others to continue on into the twilight years of their life. Just by showing up and finishing races, you'll be motivating the masses to live a healthy lifestyle, with running as a key component. Be proud of yourself and be ready to high-five your way through every workout and every race.

MATURE MECHANICS 101

How you run always matters, but frankly, as we get older, it matters even more. Maintaining proper running form may look a little different for everyone, but what it ultimately means is the same—you'll be able to keep up your distance year after year. Good running technique helps us go faster and helps protect our joints and muscles from repetitive motion over the miles.

During my coaching career, I've watched and studied thousands of runners, from newbies to world record holders, and what I've concluded is that everyone is unique in their running form. I think it's safe to assume that even the biomechanical experts out there would agree that we're all different in the way we run, as slight and subtle as those differences may be.

There are a few running methods out there that claim runners using them achieve the best technique over the years, but most of these are weighted heavily in theory and fall short on evidence. The Pose Method and ChiRunning, for example, both have one major concept in common—they assert that if we lean forward while running, then we can use gravity, the constant force that holds us to the planet, to propel ourselves forward.

There are no secrets or tricks. We are all capable of reaching our best running form by following a few simple steps.

ADJUST YOUR POSTURE

Posture, in a nutshell, is the position in which you carry your body. The coordinated actions of various muscles are required to get into—and maintain—a good posture. Your posture while sitting, standing, or running is important. All the recommended running techniques out there tout the importance of maintaining proper posture while running. I, myself, have a very upright running posture when running. I believe it's important to think about staying "tall" and "upright." Running "tall" does a couple of things—it helps keep your center of gravity right where it should be (near your navel), and it helps enhance your respiratory function by allowing for adequate rib expansion (inhalation) and contraction (exhalation) so you're able to take in more oxygen. Go ahead and try taking a deep breath while you're hunched over—it simply doesn't work.

In addition to the enhanced gas exchange touched on above, there's also a mechanical energy advantage when running upright. The Achilles tendon functions optimally when running with perfect posture.

Holding yourself up a little taller is not just great for improving your running performance, but it's also important for maintaining a healthy life and having a more balanced body. Sitting, standing, walking, and running tall does require a strong core, one that has endurance and is resistant to fatigue, but don't worry—we'll get to that in a minute.

Do a quick posture check while you are running. Look for these key variables to make sure you are maximizing your alignment:

» Your head should be up and your eyes should be looking forward as opposed to down.

» Keep your back straight.

» Shoulders should be level, relaxed.

» Don't lean forward . . . or backward.

ENGAGE YOUR CORE

When we talk about our core, the first thing most people think about is their abs. But this complex group of muscles is made up of so much more than that. Your core, which is located primarily in your belly region and back, includes these major muscle groups: pelvic floor muscles (hello, Kegels!); transverse abdominis; multifidus; internal and external obliques; rectus abdominus (six-pack); erector spinae (muscles along the vertebrae), especially the longissimus thoracis; and the diaphragm (muscle that controls breathing). Additional minor muscles that comprise your core are the lumbar (low back) muscles, quadratus lumborum,

deep rotators of the femur (upper leg bone), and the cervical muscles of the neck.

So why are these muscles important to running and the rest of your daily life? Think of your core as a bridge that connects your shoulders to your hips. Both regions of the body are important for smooth running, and they need to complement one another as you stride. Keep in mind, we run with our whole bodies, and we need the momentum from our arms to counteract the torque that is generated from our hips with every step.

Here's a little exercise to illustrate my point . . . kneel down with your knees flexed on the floor, the tops of your feet touching the floor and your bottom resting on your heels. Sit up tall, then pump your arms by your sides, like you're running. Notice that your knees move back and forth slightly as you do it, which is a direct response to the torque you're creating with your arms. This proves that the force generated in your shoulder girdle gets transmitted to your hips via your torso and can either negatively or positively impact your running form and biomechanics.

PUMP YOUR ARMS

Have you ever tried walking without moving your arms? Feels weird, right? That's because your body parts aren't designed to move independently of one another. When you're running, the role your arms play is even more critical. For one, arm movement while running is important in counterbalancing the rotational forces that our hips and legs create. But even bigger, research shows that pumping your arms simultaneously while you stride actually makes running easier. A study published in the *Journal of Experimental Biology* revealed that when runners held their arms loosely by their sides and didn't engage them while running, they experienced a 3 percent drop in their metabolic efficiency. And when the same runners held their hands on top of their heads, their running efficiency dropped a whopping 13 percent!

"Pump your arms!" My high school coach would stand at the top of a hill on our cross-country course and shout this over and over again as my team and I sprinted up a seemingly never-ending 100m dirt hill every Tuesday during the cross-country season. He wanted us to know that it was always okay to use our arms for extra momentum and to never fear doing it during a competition, especially when we were going uphill.

You always want to move your arms from your shoulder joint, and your elbow should be bent 90 degrees, so it forms a perfect right angle. If the angle is greater than 90 degrees, then your stride length will increase too much, causing you to lose efficiency. If the angle is less than 90 degrees, your stride length will shorten too much, also causing you to—you guessed it—lose efficiency. A 90-degree angle allows you to truly maximize your stride length. Think of this relationship like a pendulum and a lever.

HAVE HAPPY FEET

I have a PSA: Take care of your feet; they're special. The human foot is remarkable, and if you're a runner, it can be either your strongest—or your weakest—link. It's composed of 26 bones (33 joints) and is flimsy and floppy when not in use, but instantaneously becomes a rigid lever once weight is put on it. Genius.

Our feet endure so much every day. Once you add on the extra miles as a runner, it's no wonder we're all losing toenails, getting callouses and blisters, and experiencing other aches and pains.

There are a few easy things you can do to make your feet happier and your running smoother.

» Make sure you're wearing shoes that fit your feet properly. Everyone is different, so just because your training partner has found the perfect pair of shoes, it doesn't mean that they're also going to be perfect for you.

» Go to a local running store and have them perform a gait

analysis and proper fitting. Be sure there is enough room in the toe box to allow your toes to spread out and for your foot to swell and lengthen during long runs. Run in them before you leave the store. Remember, comfort is key.

You should perform routine maintenance on your feet as well.

» Consider it part of your regular training routine. You can even do it at night while you're winding down and watching TV. Gently spread your toes apart, flex and extend them and roll your ankles in both directions to rotate them. Stretch them.

» Grab a golf ball, place it on the floor, and gently roll the bottom of your foot on top of it. This action will stretch out the plantar fascia and help break up fibrous adhesions that have built up over the years.

Having supple and flexible feet is super important if you want to continue running pain-free year after year.

COUNT OUT YOUR CADENCE

When running, you should aim for 160 to 180 steps per minute, counting every time your left and right foot hit the ground. You can simply count in your head, or try using a GPS watch. Having a quicker landing pattern will reduce the impact forces in running and can help minimize injuries as a result.

Also, when running into a headwind, quickening and shortening your stride will ensure that you don't lose too much momentum from the wind pushing you backward. The inverse is true when you have the wind at your back: try to lengthen your stride and spend more time in the air to allow the wind to push you along.

How do you determine your cadence without a GPS watch? During a run, count the number of times your left foot strikes the ground during a 30-second time frame, and then multiply that number by four. This will give you your total amount of foot strikes per minute, or your cadence.

A friend of mine, Dr. Douglas Will, a 68-year-old neurologist and passionate athlete, insists that keeping his cadence consistent over the years is what has allowed him to run well for the last four decades. I met Doug when I was 25 years old, a fresh new coach in Mammoth Lakes. He was twice my age and had a wealth of knowledge in the sport of running. At the time, he mentioned that he still felt as fast as he did when he was in his 30s, competing in the half marathon (with a personal best of 1:18, which he reached at 38) and marathon. He said his cadence has been relatively the same through the decades and he feels the only reason he's slowing down is because of lower power output from his legs.

ASSESSING YOUR FORM

Now that you know how important it is to maintain good form, it's time to learn how to assess where you currently are. Ever take a glimpse of yourself when you're running past a storefront window, checking yourself out in the reflection? Did you think, "I look good!" or maybe it was more like, "Is that seriously what I look like when I run?!"

HOW CAN I ASSESS MY FORM?

A running form assessment can be valuable, and it's honestly one of the tools I use all the time with the elite runners I coach. Biomechanists and local coaches can analyze your form (there are human performance labs that are set up to do it) with treadmills and computer software that can measure degrees of joint flexion, along with your horizontal and vertical planes of motion. The best way to do a self-assessment is to record a video of yourself running on a treadmill.

Everyone has a camera on their phone. Ask a friend or relative to take a video of you. But if you really don't want an audience, simply place your phone in a position where you can capture the video yourself. There are several apps that are designed to analyze running form, so you can download one to your phone, upload your video, and get feedback quickly.

In all likelihood, if your form feels good and you're not experiencing any running-related aches and pains, then it's probably "sound" and doesn't need much improving. Some things to check for though: See if your head is over your shoulders or protracted in a forward position. Check out those arms. What are they doing? Are your elbows at a 90-degree angle or close to it? Do your wrists break (when they go limp and flex on your back swing)? You want to avoid that, as it wastes energy and throws a hiccup in your stride frequency optimization, so keep a straight wrist. One thing that helps is to imagine you're holding something delicate in your hand that you don't want to squish.

Now, take a look at what your head is doing. Is it directly over your shoulders? Meaning, are your ears in line with the tops of your shoulders? If so, great! You're doing it right. If your head is slightly protracted forward, then this could pose a problem toward the end of long runs, or when you're building up your mileage for a longer race. This positioning changes your center of gravity and causes you to place more of your mass out in front of you, which in turn puts excess stress on your posterior muscles, or everything on your backside (glutes, hamstrings, calves). This, unfortunately, causes more stress on your tendons, and I personally believe it's the root of many calf strains and Achilles and plantar injuries. Remember, run tall.

LISTEN TO YOUR BODY

Every runner should be able to finish an easy recovery run feeling fresh, like you could do the entire distance again. It should leave you feeling renewed and invigorated. It's always a good idea to do a quick check-in with yourself after an easy run. If you're feeling okay or even better than when you started, in all likelihood, your form is sound and functioning well.

One question I'm asked a lot is if you should modify your form when training and racing different distances, and the quick answer is YES. However, there's a *but*. (There's almost always a "but.") If you were to do a one-mile road race (which I highly recommend if you haven't done one before—they're a blast!), your arm swing would be more forceful, with your hand

WHAT TO PUT ON YOUR FEET (OR NOT)

If you've been running through the decades like I have, you're probably pretty particular about what type of shoes you run in. Many of my athletes are creatures of habit, and they stick with the shoes they've been running in for years and years simply because they know they work and they're not getting injured. But every now and then, shoe companies change up their designs, color schemes, materials used, and they change the shoe so much that it doesn't work for some runners anymore—so then what? I am a big advocate of heading down to your local running store and asking the experts, the ones who sell shoes to runners of all ages and abilities on a daily basis. You're very likely to learn something new and potentially find a new favorite pair of shoes.

There are many perfect shoes out there for every runner. The major shoe companies sink millions of dollars into research and development each year to make a wide variety of shoes that work well for all different types of feet and foot strike patterns. I also learned that the people who work at local running stores are passionate about running and legitimately want to improve every runner's experience out there on the road and trails.

In the mid-2000s, a barefoot running craze swept the world. Running shoe companies started making their own versions of a minimalist shoe, the closest thing to being barefoot they could offer. Many of them looked like gloves for your feet, with just a thin layer of rubber on the bottom to protect your sole from debris. The theory was that since our ancestors ran barefoot, they didn't have medial posting to correct overpronation, and they didn't get injured all the time, then clearly there was something to it or something to that effect.

But the reality is, if you're training for a 10K or longer, your feet need shoes to train and race in. Sure, our running mechanics are slightly different, possibly even better when we are barefoot, but most of us, growing up in Western society, all wore shoes our entire lives. So now we need the cushioning and support that well-engineered shoes bring to the game. If you're reading this book, then you're likely training at a fairly high level, logging 30 to 60 miles per week, and maybe running half-marathons and marathons every year. This level of training is extraordinarily difficult on the body, and it's above and beyond what the other 99 percent of people on the planet are doing. With marathon training, you're asking your body to endure a stressful training regimen. For this, you need to protect your body and protect your feet from the impact forces of repetitively striking the ground.

coming up higher at the end of the forward swing and your elbow pushing farther behind you on the back swing. Your back kick (when your heel comes off the ground) would be higher, and you would pull your foot through the leg swing cycle much more forcefully. And your knee lift would be higher, as you want your stride length to be near its maximum. But most of us are not racing one mile these days, at least not often enough to try switching our form for the occasion.

AVOIDING COMMON INJURIES

We all want to avoid injuries, especially as we get older and recovery takes longer.

For starters, I've got a few simple rules you can follow:

1. **Stay hydrated.** Avoid excessive caffeine and alcohol consumption. Most musculoskeletal injuries are caused by not consuming enough electrolytes or drinking enough water. Consuming too much caffeine can also make you dehydrated and put you at risk of cramps and strains that are far too typical in training.

2. **Stretch.** Do this periodically throughout the day, even if it's just for a few minutes.

3. **Warm up.** Simply start every run off at a very, very slow pace. Heck, start off walking for five minutes, so you can allow your body to warm up gradually and naturally. Some days it might take five to ten minutes to ease into your average pace—other days it might take 45!

4. **Listen to your body.** I repeat, LISTEN TO YOUR BODY. No one else can hear what's happening in there. If something is sore, don't run through it. Missing one or two runs to allow a body part to calm down will benefit you in the long run. Your goal is to stay healthy enough to run another day.

5. **Ease your transitions.** Most of us sit . . . a lot. This nonaction is what causes most injuries. Trying to immediately transition to running from this sedentary position takes the body by surprise, and it may reject the activity. This is why you need to take your time transitioning from either sleeping for eight hours or sitting for a few to doing a workout or run. Remember to listen to your body and never force it through anything. It's a common practice for Kenyan runners to start their runs with a walk. I've been to world championships and

Olympic Games and watched speedy Team Kenya start a hard training session with a slow 10-minute group walk. If they can slow down, so can you!

TEN COMMON RUNNING-RELATED INJURIES

Type of Injury: Stress Fracture

CAUSE: This small crack in any weight-bearing bone is usually found in the tibia, fibula, femur, pelvis, and metatarsal. Repetitive trauma to those bones is usually caused by the impact forces that occur when landing during walking and running. It could also be surface-related if you're running on cement or pavement too much, but the most common cause is increasing your training load too quickly or adding in speed training while simultaneously increasing training volume.

EARLY SIGNS: A dull ache or burning sensation in the affected area. Consult an orthopedic doctor about getting an MRI. If caught early enough (in the stress reaction stage, not broken through yet), the downtime from weight-bearing activity can be cut in half. If the MRI comes back showing a slight crack, then it's likely the doctor will prescribe a walking cast or put you on crutches for six to eight weeks.

HOW TO PREVENT AND TREAT: Eat a robust diet filled with foods rich in vitamin D and calcium. Wear shoes that are cushioned enough to absorb the impact forces of running. Stick to a sensible running routine, adding miles gradually and safely to your training (about a 10 percent increase each week, with a reduction week every three weeks to allow for recovery). Consult your doctor about taking vitamin D and calcium supplements for your bones as well.

Type of Injury: IT Band Syndrome (ITBS)

CAUSE: An exact cause is not really known, but experts have concluded that old shoes (with too many miles on them) could be at least partly to blame, as they can change the way your foot strikes the ground. Another possible cause is running on a cambered or sloped road, which can throw off your hip height and lead to an imbalance. I personally think that another possible cause is starting multiple runs in a dehydrated state, which leads to subtle muscle cramping in your hips and tightens up vulnerable muscles and tendons.

EARLY SIGNS: A sharp pain on the outside (lateral aspect) of your knee. This sharp pain is usually felt when your knee is bent beyond 20 to 30 degrees. A runner will likely feel this sensation just a mile or two into their training run.

HOW TO PREVENT AND TREAT:
Stay hydrated and eat well. Replace your shoes frequently (every 250 to 300 miles). Also, start each of your runs off slowly, allowing your body to gradually warm up. And be sure you activate those hip adductors, or groin muscles, before you run. Stand tall and squeeze your legs together until they feel fatigued. This little exercise will help wake up those oft-forgotten muscles and get them working before breaking into a sprint. This group of muscles opposes the muscles that control your IT band of fascia that's hurting your knee. By activating the adductors (the muscles used to bring your knees together), the abductors (the muscles used to widen your stance) tend to relax and loosen up, which allows your IT band to have a little bit of slack so it doesn't rub against the bony part of the outside of your knee.

Type of Injury: Achilles Tendonitis

CAUSE: Worn-out shoes and tight calves or weak/tight hip flexors and restricted ankle mobility. Starting speed work too aggressively can contribute to this injury as well. Dehydration can also cause tight calves, which can lead to the irritation of your Achilles tendon (the largest and thickest tendon in the body). Tight hip flexors (often from sitting too much) can lead to Achilles irritation and eventually tendonitis,

too. If your hip flexors are not working properly, then the calves have to make up for it in a more forceful way. Too much uphill running can also lead to a sore Achilles.

EARLY SIGNS: Soreness and pain in the tendon itself, either right at the insertion point or as high as two to three inches above the heel bone (calcaneus).

HOW TO PREVENT AND TREAT:
Work on maintaining good ankle flexibility, stretch your calves frequently throughout the day, start each run off slowly, and stay hydrated. To treat this injury, you'll need to stop running altogether. Perform eccentric calf lowering exercises off a step with your injured leg. Elevate and ice lightly, for no more than ten minutes at a time. Avoid running uphill until the pain subsides.

Type of Injury: Runner's Knee (Patellofemoral Pain Syndrome)

CAUSE: Tight quadriceps muscles can cause a dull pain surrounding the kneecap.

EARLY SIGNS: You'll feel discomfort about one or two miles into a run, usually like a dull ache behind or above your kneecap. The pain does not go away and will likely prevent you from running any farther.

HOW TO PREVENT AND TREAT:

Hydrate! Stretch your quadriceps well every day, either before or after running. Perform a set of squats (without weight) a few times a week to strengthen this muscle group, too—I'll give you more details on how to do this in chapter 3.

Type of Injury: High Hamstring Tendinopathy

CAUSE: This injury usually starts off very small and with little discomfort but is usually ignored and then worsens over a period of weeks and months. Again, I believe dehydration is a major cause.

EARLY SIGNS: The pain associated with this injury is located at the very top of the hamstring and just below the buttocks. If you bend over to touch your toes and feel a sharp grab in this location, then it's likely there is damage to the area. Very slow running with a short stride seems to be fine, but if your pace quickens and your stride lengthens, there will be severe discomfort.

HOW TO PREVENT AND TREAT:

Stay hydrated. Avoid sitting for long periods of time. Stretch your hamstrings for a few minutes every day. Get a massage to increase blood flow. Ice the area occasionally until your symptoms are gone. Avoid a long stride when running.

Type of Injury: Black (or Lost) Toenails

CAUSE: When training for a long-distance event such as a marathon, our feet have a tendency to swell and lengthen as they fatigue. If your shoes are too small, your toes will start to bash into the front of the toe box, causing irritation to your nails.

EARLY SIGNS: Sore toes, right at the tips. You'll possibly see some discoloration after just one run. If your toes are black, it means that blood has collected underneath your nail(s).

HOW TO PREVENT AND TREAT:

Trim your toenails frequently, once or twice a week. Purchase shoes that have plenty of room in the toe box so your toes have ample space to swell during a long run. I've heard of runners having their toenails surgically removed so this doesn't happen to them, but that's an extreme, totally unnecessary way to address this issue if you ask me.

Type of Injury: Plantar Fasciitis

CAUSE: Chronic dehydration plus tight calves and hip flexors are likely to blame.

EARLY SIGNS: Pain in the plantar fascia is usually felt when you first start walking around in the morning. The bottom of your heel feels sore and tender to the touch. The discomfort can disappear in the first few minutes of your run, but the pain starts to linger longer and longer after a few weeks.

HOW TO PREVENT AND TREAT:

Make sure you stretch your calves and hip flexors well each day. Stay hydrated during long training runs. Ice the affected area for 10 minutes a couple of times every day. Frequent calf massages can also help loosen the tension pulling up on your arch.

Type of Injury: Shin Splints

CAUSE: Worn out shoes and/or increasing training volume too quickly is likely the culprit.

EARLY SIGNS: Pain is felt on the medial side of your tibia bone. It's caused by inflammation of your muscle and tendon, which are ever so slightly tearing away from the bone. The inside of your shin will feel sore when running.

HOW TO PREVENT AND TREAT:

Check the wear on your shoes and keep a tally on how many miles you've logged, changing them out before they're completely broken down (250 to 300 miles). Add mileage into your schedule slowly and methodically, with no more than a 10 to 15 percent increase from week to week. To treat, you'll need rest or a severe reduction in mileage, icing, and light massage.

Type of Injury: Patellar Tendonitis

CAUSE: The mechanism behind this injury is roughly the same as runner's knee, but the symptoms are different. Inflammation in this area is brought on by tight quads and a great deal of pounding on the roads, especially if you're doing a lot of downhill running. Chances are, you have been feeling pain for a while but have been ignoring the signs and/or running with a cheap knee brace, trying to make it better.

EARLY SIGNS: Lower knee pain when running. This injury seems to be more common in men.

HOW TO PREVENT AND TREAT:

Keep your training progression easy and methodical. At the first signs of pain at the bottom of your kneecap, take a day or two off. Get a massage and apply ice to the affected area for up to 10 minutes each day. Do a quick check of your current training shoes to see if there is excessive wear and tear.

Type of Injury: Blisters

CAUSE: Friction between the skin on your feet and your socks, often due to an ill-fitting shoe. Wearing the wrong socks or not breaking in shoes enough before going for a longer-distance training run can also cause irritation. Blisters on your toes can be caused by a shoe that is too small for you.

EARLY SIGNS: A rubbing or pinching pain on the skin of your feet in one or more spots that causes you to change your stride pattern to seek relief.

HOW TO PREVENT AND TREAT: Run in shoes that fit your feet well and choose socks that provide enough coverage and support. If blisters persist, you can rub some Vaseline on your feet to reduce the friction of your sock against your skin. Do not pop a blister, as opening it could lead to an infection. When not running, wear sandals to let air get to the affected skin. Use a Band-Aid to cover and protect the area if your training needs to continue.

COMPLEMENTARY PRACTICES

Let's cover activities that mix up both training and recovery goals for the runner. We talked about avoiding injuries in the previous section, so I'll reiterate here that our bodies need some variety to avoid repetitive stress injuries and to recover fully.

In an effort to run successfully (read: injury-free) for decades, we must incorporate more than just running into our weekly routines. Adding in strength training, stretching, yoga, walking or hiking, and some interval training sessions will help prevent boredom and improve your overall fitness and running performance. Mixing things up will also reduce your risk of injury and aid in your recovery.

STRENGTH TRAINING

It has been known for decades that strength or resistance training can enhance endurance. Strength training is a broad category and many folks often get confused about how to apply these types of exercises and movements into their running regimen. I always try to break it down into simple and basic components for my athletes, so it feels approachable and easy to execute.

First off, know that a little strength work can go a long way, and you don't have to use heavy weights. Etching out 15 to 20 minutes, two to three times a week, is really all you need to do. During each training session, your goal should be to hit all of the major muscle groups in your body—your quads, hips, abs, back, and shoulders. Try to squeeze in a couple exercises for your arms and shoulders, such as push-ups or dumbbell overhead presses; a couple for your legs, like walking lunges or squats; and a couple for your core, such as alternating side planks or Supermans.

Adding a weightlifting component into your current training program will bring big benefits. For one, your tendons, ligaments, muscle tissue, and bones all become stronger and more resistant to injury. This is especially good as we get older and have to start worrying about things like osteopenia (a weakening of bone tissue).

Strength training also helps create balance in your body, which becomes increasingly essential as we age. It's common for us runners to become unbalanced, either from sustaining an injury or just running on the same cambered sidewalk for months on end. It's important to be intent on creating balance when you are lifting weights or performing core exercises.

When performing resistance exercises, keep in mind that less is more. If you're just starting out, keep the weights light and perform the movements slowly and with purpose. Be sure to warm up lightly beforehand, too, getting your heart pumping and muscles moving with a short, easy run either outside the gym or on a treadmill. When you're finished lifting, cool down with light aerobic work to flush out some soreness that you'll inevitably experience in the first few weeks.

STRETCHING AND YOGA

For the last decade, the benefits of stretching have been widely debated. I personally like to stretch afterward. I do not wish to confuse stretching with yoga though. My motto is: Stretch for performance, and do yoga to enhance the spirit, along with the mind-body connection. Both can be valuable and positive training components when gearing up for a race.

My wife, Deena, and I have been practicing Active Isolated Stretching (AIS) for the past 20 years for workouts and race preparation. AIS is a controlled, dynamic way of stretching muscle groups individually. You can find out more about this technique in my first book, *Running Your First Marathon,* or online by searching for "Active Isolated Stretching with the Whartons."

Stretching periodically throughout the day helps speed up recovery by allowing your muscles to return to their resting length, which helps promote blood flow to each and every muscle fiber. Years (err, decades!) of the repetitive pounding that comes with running contributes to the inevitable accumulation of scar tissue between your muscle fibers. Stretching helps break up these adhesions, or as massage therapists like to call them, "knots." If you, like most nonelite runners, can't see a massage therapist every few days, then invest in a foam roller and roll out the major muscle groups in your legs regularly. Combined with your body weight, this device breaks up the fascia between your skin and muscles to alleviate tension and assist in regaining your mobility.

Now let's talk about yoga. I get asked all the time about the benefits of yoga on running performance. I am a big supporter of yoga for any athlete, to be honest. I believe yoga can teach all of us how to have better body awareness through guided sessions with an instructor. I do like to emphasize that performing yoga should be for the sake of getting better at yoga and not to become a better runner. View yoga as a way to calm your mind and harness the focus that leads to being productive. By balancing your physical being with your mental being, you'll fall into alignment fairly easily before your next training session. The best runners in the world aren't necessarily doing yoga, but they work on their flexibility and mobility every day during their training. These athletes have learned how to be present and focused from years of experience; they know how to get their minds and bodies to peak at the right time every day, week, and season. The rest of us, well, we could probably use a little more help in that department. So if time allows

in your weekly schedule, try a few guided yoga sessions and see what you think.

WALKING AND HIKING

The next best thing to a daily run is a daily walk or hike. No question. Many of the Japanese elite distance runners employ walking into their training. It's a great mode of recovery that's low impact and will get your heart rate up enough to circulate the blood through your veins and arteries, helping flush out the metabolic waste produced from training runs. This can be a really productive way to recover mentally and physically after a tough training event or race.

Hiking is also a wonderful way to get out into nature and explore a new trail that you've never experienced before. You can take mental notes on what it would be like to come back and run the trail, or take a stab at the climb or rocky descent. If you're into ultra-marathon racing, hiking is a normal part of the race strategy, too. Ever see someone in a trail race with their hands on the tops of their thighs, pushing down on them with every power step they take up a steep grade? Yep, this is a useful strategy!

Walking is a great way to warm up before a workout or a race. It is also a smart way to get in a little aerobic work when recovering from a hard event or building back fitness from some time off due to an injury or illness. Many elite athletes who have been injured work themselves up to walking for an hour with no pain before they try a training run.

INTERVAL TRAINING

Interval training is a key component to maximizing your running performance. It's essentially alternating hard efforts with easy efforts—and it can be applied to both strength and running workouts alike. Some interval workouts are designed with specific race demands in mind, like running 6 x 800m (½ mile) with a two-minute recovery between each. The 800m portions are supposed to be run at goal 5K pace, as 6 x 800m is roughly 5K worth of work. Another example of interval training that has a wider set of parameters is that of a natural fartlek, the kind of run that I find myself on at the beginning of each season. After about two to three weeks of aerobic base training, I find myself slowly picking up the pace and accelerating for several minutes, then backing off to a slow jog again. Each hard bout of running lasts somewhere between one and three minutes, followed by one to three minutes of easy running to allow for recovery, and this pattern continues for the entirety of my 60-minute run.

What are the benefits of interval training? It's been well proven that a quick 30-second sprint can boost human growth hormone (HGH) production by over 500 percent. Men and women all produce HGH, a wonderful molecule that floats around the body repairing damaged tissues, rebuilding them to be stronger and better than before. We need a steady diet of intervals to keep us fit, fast, and healthy.

Here's a simple workout to get started—you don't need a track, just a watch with a timer: Do a 20-minute warm-up running easily, followed by a few light, dynamic stretches. Then run one minute at 5K race pace, jog for a minute, and repeat. Do 8 to 12 reps. Run easily for a few minutes to cool down. And you're all done . . . high-five! You can eventually take this workout to the track and run 8 to 12 x 400m (one lap around the track), with a one- to two-minute recovery interval between each. Try to incorporate this into your routine once a week.

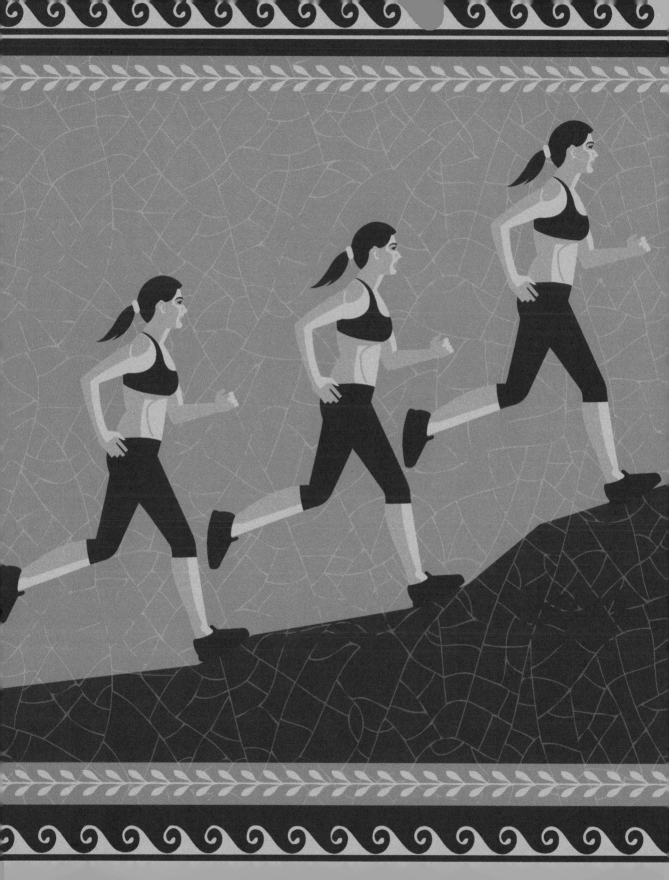

CHAPTER THREE

PERSPIRATION

HOW TO BUILD A RUNNER'S BODY

We run with our whole body. Keep this in mind when you're training and while reading this book. If any body part isn't working at 100 percent, then we're not the most optimized versions of ourselves. So how can we all work toward reaching that 100 percent and striding toward the goal of optimization? Rather than thinking about your entire body at once, focus on making smaller, more manageable improvements one at a time. After scanning yourself from head to toe, create a checklist for restrictions and limitations. Now, devise a plan to tackle each of the items on your list, incorporating exercises to enhance mobility, stability, and strength in the places you need them most. Each of these elements will help prevent injury and put you on the path to becoming bulletproof in your training for decades to come.

In this chapter, I'll share exercises and movements with you that are designed specifically to build the mobility, stability, and strength required to keep running at your best, no matter your age. Mobility is defined as "the ability to move or be moved freely and easily." Just think about the 33 joints in your foot—if you had enhanced mobility in this area, you'd be able to bounce out of bed and hit the road running immediately. And stability keeps us all on our feet, steadying our every move so we don't fall over constantly. It's defined as "the ability to maintain control of joint movement or position by coordinating actions of surrounding tissues and the neuromuscular system."

EXERCISES FOR MOBILITY, STABILITY, AND INJURY PREVENTION

POSTURE

SHOULDER PASS-THROUGHS

Shoulder pass-throughs are fantastic for improving the range of motion in your shoulders. The movement helps lengthen your muscles and tendons that surround and support the shoulder girdle. Also, by stretching out the pectoral muscles in your chest, you'll be able to reposition your shoulder much easier into a retracted position, which helps maintain an upright posture.

BENEFITS: Removes tension from the muscles that act upon your shoulder joints, allowing your arms to move more freely—and be less restricted—during your runs. Loose and free-flowing shoulders will translate to free-flowing hips, as well. An added benefit to this exercise: It can help open up your ribs and improve your lung capacity and breathing by stretching the muscles that act upon the ribcage.

HOW TO:

1. Hold a PVC pipe (approximately four feet long), with an overhand grip that is slightly wider than your shoulders.

2. Keeping a slight bend in your elbows, slowly lift the pipe directly overhead, and lower it down your backside.

3. Do about 10 reps of this exercise once a day to see results.

For bonus mobility benefits, explore different angles with your body when you're moving through the motion. For example, rotate your torso or raise one hand higher than the other when moving the pipe.

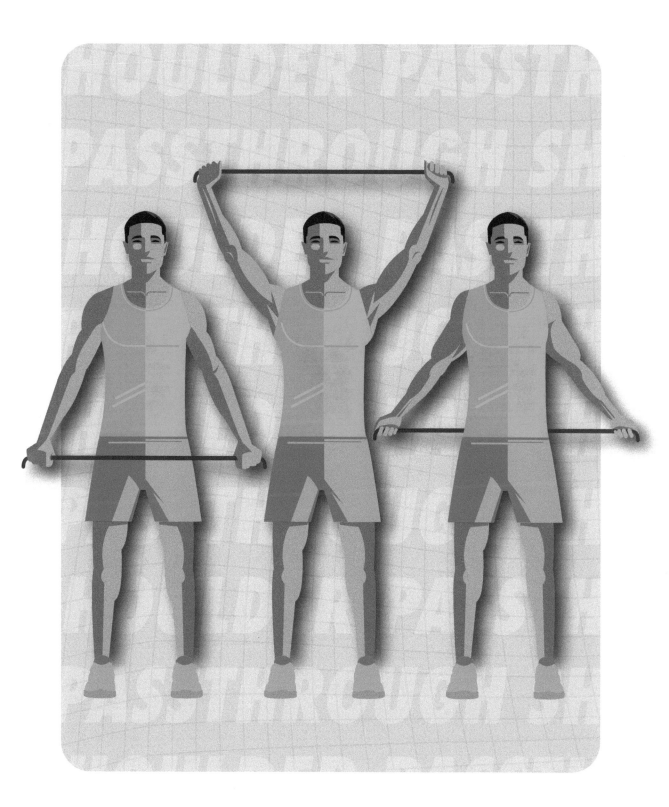

ISOMETRIC ROWS

The primary muscles that work to maintain good posture in your upper body are the rhomboideus and trapezius muscle groups. These can become weak and stretched out with the daily rigors of typing on a computer or sitting in the car too long. This exercise is used to turn on inactive back and shoulder muscles that might lay dormant the rest of the day.

BENEFITS: Pulling your shoulders back will help keep your head over your shoulders, rather than that undesired protracted forward position we discussed in chapter 2. It can also help alleviate posterior neck pain and build overall strength that you need to stay upright, or nice and tall, when you're running.

HOW TO:

1. Sit in a chair with your back tall, feet flat on floor, and shoulders down and relaxed.

2. Bend your elbows into a 90-degree angle by your sides. Draw both elbows back until your hands are by your ribs and squeeze your shoulder blades together; hold for 10 seconds. Be sure to breathe throughout this isometric contraction.

3. Return to starting position. Recover for a few seconds and repeat. Continue for one minute in total.

Perform this exercise a few times a day.

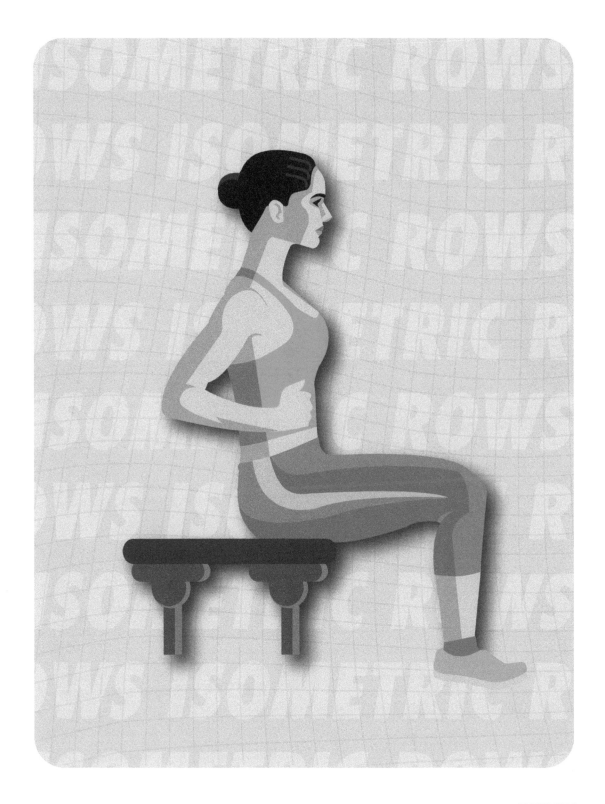

COBRA POSE FOR BACK EXTENSION

We spend so much time hunched over, leaning, or bending forward and so little time bending over backward. In time, we become stiff and slowly lose the ability to extend our spines, which can lead to all kinds of awkward movement patterns and injuries. This move stretches out your abdominal muscles while simultaneously strengthening your erector spinae muscles, which support the spine.

BENEFITS: Prevent that unwanted slouch that somehow slowly creeps its way into our lives by doing this exercise once a day. This move is not just for the back—it also improves blood flow to the abdominal region, assisting in the nourishment of its tissues.

HOW TO:

1. Lie face down on the floor, with your hands directly under your shoulders, and your legs extended behind you.

2. Inhale, and then on your next exhale, slowly press into your palms, extending your arms and lifting your head and chest off the floor. This will cause your back to arch slightly, so try to relax. Be sure to keep your pelvis on the ground throughout.

3. Lift your chest as high as comfortable while still breathing through the movement.

4. Hold your highest position for 3 seconds, and then gently lower back to start, placing your chest and head back on the floor.

5. Do 3 to 5 reps, trying to lift your chest and head a little bit (1 percent) higher each time.

If you find this exercise challenging, that's okay. Be patient—it will get easier over time.

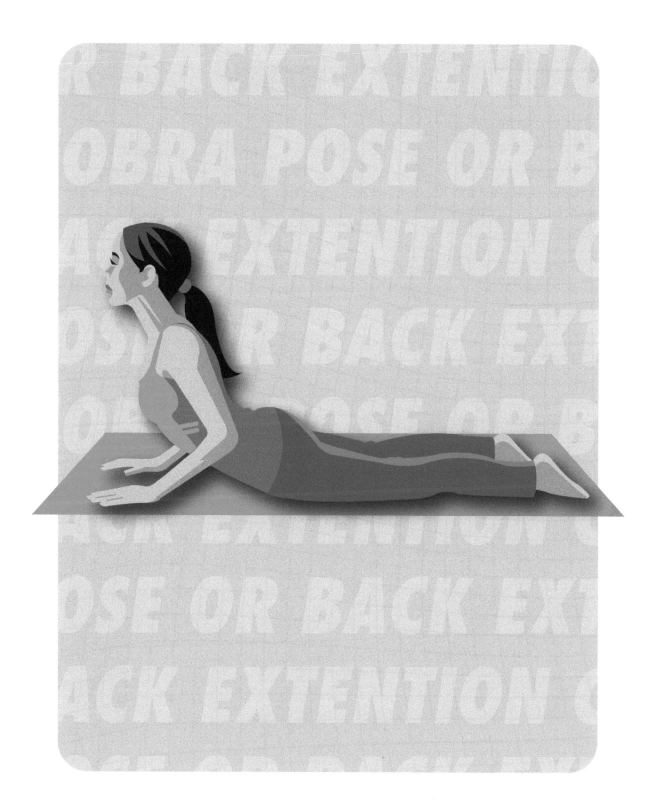

CORE

SUPERMAN

This exercise engages your back muscles, shoulders, glutes, and hamstrings. By default, most runners don't have great strength in this area due to a lack of muscular demand on your backside when running, which is why this exercise is such a helpful tool for turning on and recruiting these muscles.

BENEFITS: Performing this exercise a few times every week will help create balance between your abdominal flexors (abs) and your back extensors. Since there are no weights involved, all resistance comes from gravity and the tension in your body. This exercise might feel particularly challenging at first, due to all that tension and weakness in your back, but be patient and take it slowly.

1. Lie face down on the floor, with your arms stretched overhead and your legs together and extended behind you. Simultaneously lift your head, chest, arms, and legs a few inches off the floor, keeping your neck and shoulders relaxed, your abs engaged, and your legs together.

2. Remember to breathe. You're calling upon a vast number of muscle cells to perform these movements and they need oxygen.

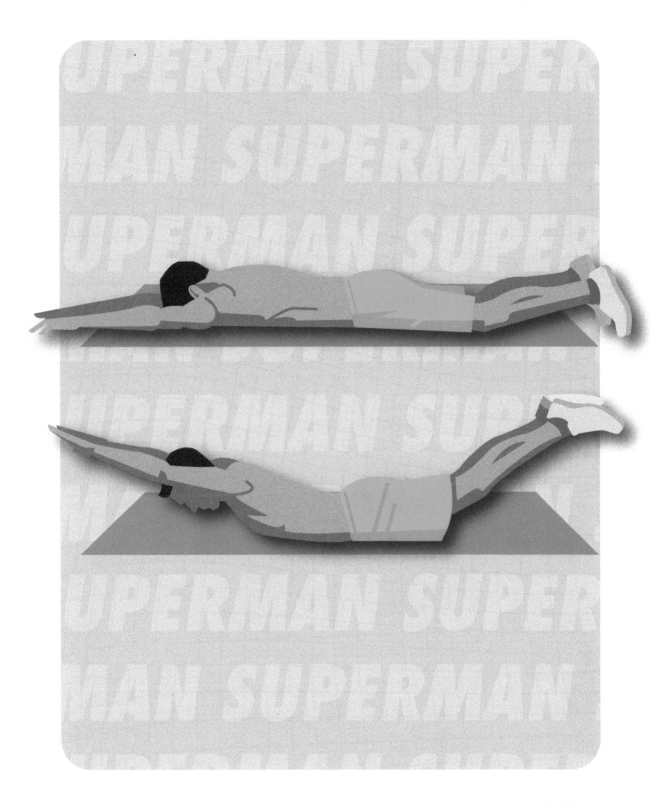

FOREARM PLANK WITH VARIATIONS

We're all familiar with planks. Planks are a type of isometric contraction, which is basically an exercise that involves contracting—or tensing up—your muscles without moving a joint. I'm not a believer in crunches or sit-ups for improving running performance because they're not functional movements—we never flex our core muscles in the same manner as in those exercises. Planks, on the other hand, are easy on your joints, particularly the vertebral ones in your back, and great for developing strength in a more natural position, similar to what we use when we run.

BENEFITS: It protects your back. The joints in your back and the muscles that surround the bones of your spine, ribs, scapula, and pelvis are necessary for propelling us forward when we walk and run.

HOW TO:

1. Lie face down on the floor (or mat) with your elbows under your shoulders, your forearms (and palms) flat on the floor, and your legs extended behind you, about hip-width apart.

2. Tuck your toes under and slowly lift your body a few inches off the floor with toes and forearms, keeping the abs engaged and back flat. Your body should form a straight—board stiff!—line from shoulders to toes.

3. If you're new to this exercise, simply hold this position for about 10 seconds, lower gently back to start, rest for 20 to 30 seconds, and repeat.

4. Continue doing forearm planks for 2 to 3 minutes total.

Once you've mastered the forearm plank, try a regular plank (with hands flat on floor directly under shoulders, rather than on your forearms).

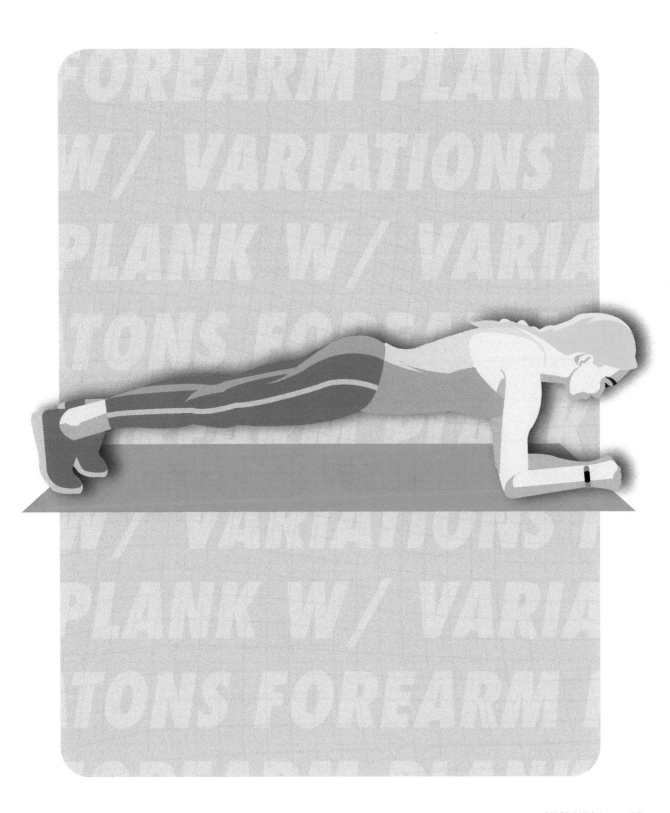

GLUTE BRIDGES

This move is great for strengthening your lower back and glutes. Glute activation is directly related to stride length, as it determines how far back your legs go when you're in full hip extension. Many older runners have the tendency to slow down over the years, do less speed work, and less maximal or near-maximal running. Glute bridges regain that lost strength by forcing you to engage and contract those muscles maximally.

BENEFITS: Erases the "spending every day behind a desk" syndrome we all seem to have. When we sit for long periods of time, we have a tendency to get stuck in that position. We can reverse the tightness by consciously engaging in purposeful exercises like—you guessed it—bridges.

HOW TO:

1. Lie face up on the floor with your knees bent, feet flat on floor, and your arms extended by your sides.

2. Now slowly lift your pelvis off the floor until you form a straight diagonal line from your knees to your shoulders.

3. Engage your abs and contract your glutes.

4. Hold this position for 2 to 3 seconds, breathing consciously throughout the movement, and then slowly lower back to start.

5. Do 10 to 20 reps.

For best results, incorporate this into your training routine two to three times each week.

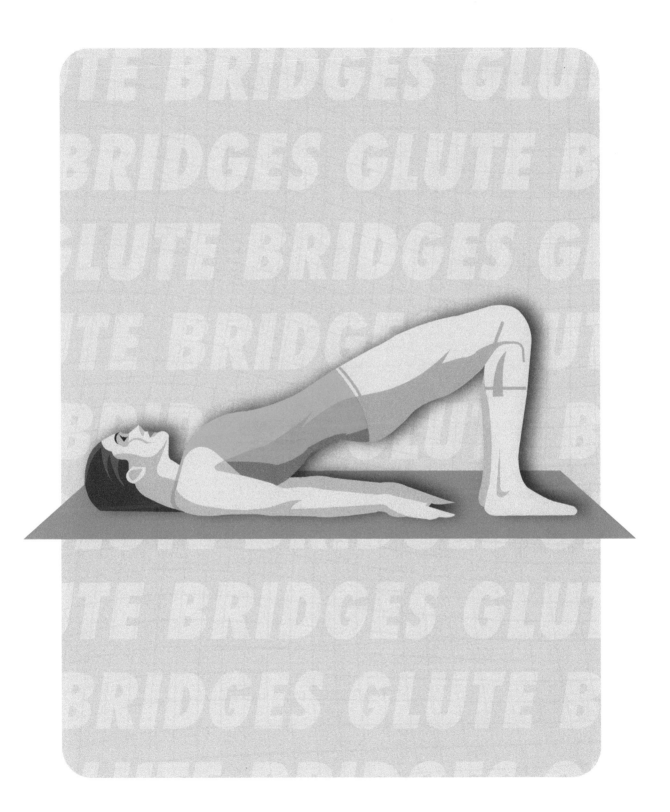

UPPER BODY

PUSH-UPS

This is a classic, and I know you've done them before, but when done correctly, they're an effective way to strengthen a lot of muscle groups (basically your entire core and upper body) all at once. I like exercises that involve 50 percent or more of your body's muscles, because they're a great use of time and super-functional. With push-ups, you'll activate all core muscles, and your shoulders, hips, and everything else down to your shins, since you're positioned on your toes.

BENEFITS: For starters, you'll increase bone density in your arms and wrist bones. Did you know that it takes approximately 1/10 of the force needed to break a bone to make it stronger? Ask yourself, if you trip while running, will the bones in your hands, wrists, and arms resist a break? Push-ups help prevent you from ever actually having to discover the answer to that question.

1. Lie face down on the floor with your hands directly under your shoulders, your abs engaged, your legs together and extended behind you, toes tucked under.

2. Press into your palms and lift your body straight up, keeping your shoulders down and trying to maintain a straight line throughout; lower back to start and repeat.

3. Begin with 5 to 10 reps, but do as many as possible. If you need to modify this and go down on your knees, that's fine. Remember, just by attempting this exercise you are making progress.

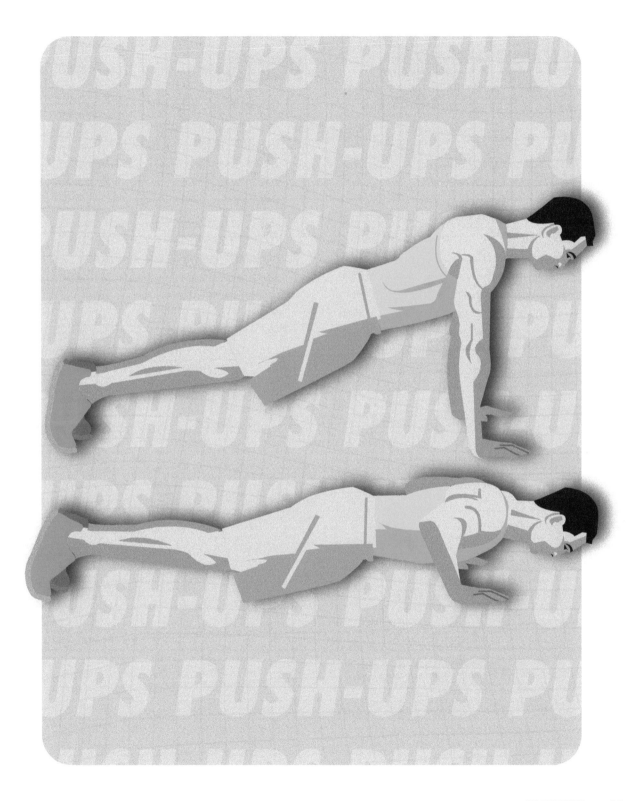

RUNNING ARMS WITH DUMBBELLS

Yes, this exercise is just like it sounds. It's not only super-specific to running, but it also acts as a core exercise.

BENEFITS: Arm and shoulder fatigue late in a race or a long run is a real thing—swinging your arms for an hour, two hours, or four-plus hours can be extremely tiring, and this move can help prevent that fatigue from setting in too early. When powering uphill or shifting gears to hit a tempo, maintaining strong momentum with your arms is hugely valuable.

1. Stand in an athletic stance with your feet shoulder-width apart, knees slightly bent, holding a light (1- to 3-pound) dumbbell in each hand, bending your arms 90 degrees at your sides.

2. Engage your abs and swing your arms back and forth, keeping your hips facing forward and abs engaged, as if you're running.

When you do this, you can really feel your core working to maintain your position right over your feet.

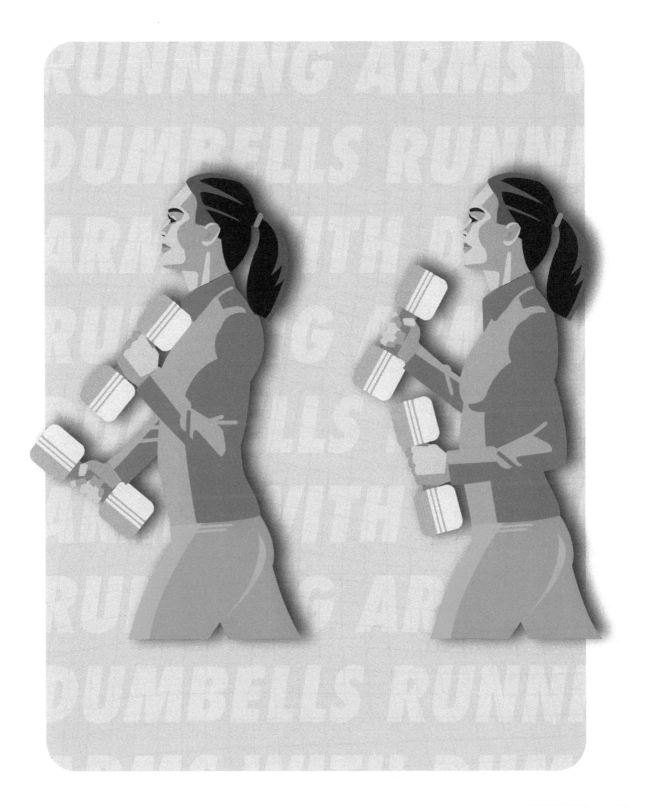

OVERHEAD PRESS

When we stimulate large amounts of muscle at once, like this move does, we get a surge of human growth hormone that helps rebuild not only the muscles we're actively stimulating, but also any other muscles that have been torn down and need restoration. The pectoralis muscles, deltoids, and triceps are all in play with this exercise.

BENEFITS: Overhead presses add stress to the bones of your arms and wrists while working in a different plane of motion than push-ups. You'll continue to build lean muscle and power in the upper body, while also supporting your shoulders and building strength that can assist them when placed in potentially compromised positions during your daily activities.

HOW TO:

You can perform this move sitting or standing, but I personally prefer standing, as more of our core stabilizers come into play.

1. Stand with your feet shoulder-width apart, knees slightly bent. Hold a medium-size barbell or dumbbells in each hand and extend your arms in front of your body, palms facing out.

2. Bend your elbows to bring the weights up to your shoulders, and then press up to fully extend your arms overhead.

3. Hold for one second, then lower back to start.

4. Do 10 to 12 reps, take a short break, and then do one more set.

This exercise can be done every day that you run.

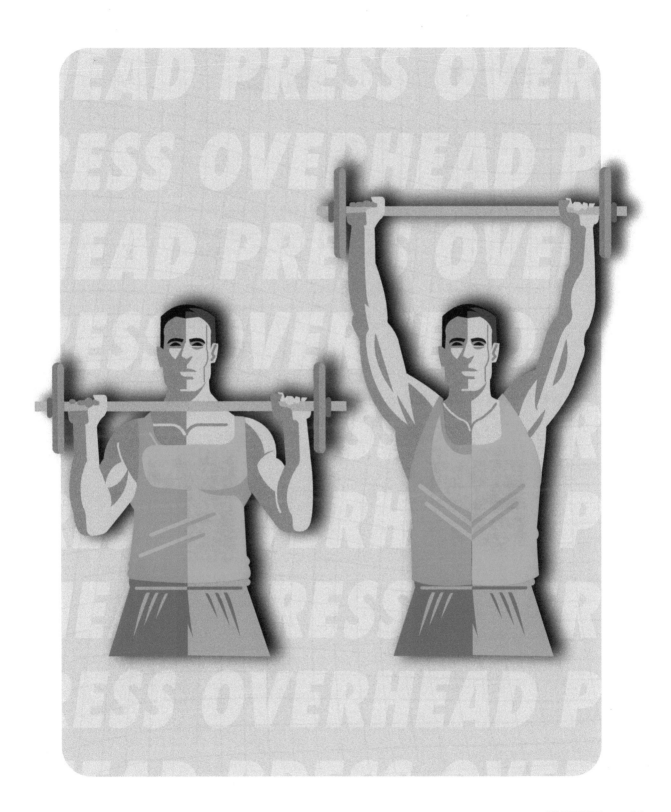

LOWER BODY

WALKING LUNGES

This exercise is fantastic not only for developing strength in your legs, but also for strengthening your core. Balance is a key component of this exercise, along with creating flexibility in your hip flexors. Performing walking lunges after sitting most of the day can be extremely valuable in preserving a strong and healthy back, while also eliminating tension in your hip flexors.

BENEFITS: Because this exercise requires a large range of motion in your hip joints, it provides a chance for your body to push and pull through a near full range of your stride length, thus making you much more efficient at all paces. By reducing tension in your hip flexors, you're able to lengthen your stride at roughly the same metabolic rate, which translates to an increased pace while running.

HOW TO:

1. Stand tall with your feet shoulder-width apart, your arms by your sides.

2. Engage your abs and take a big step forward, bending both knees to 90-degree angles, keeping your knees behind your toes.

3. Push off your back foot, bringing your knee high in front of you, and then take another big step, or lunge, forward.

4. Continue lunging forward for a total of 10 to 12 steps on each foot.

Remember, keep your core muscles activated and tight—this will help maintain your balance throughout the movement.

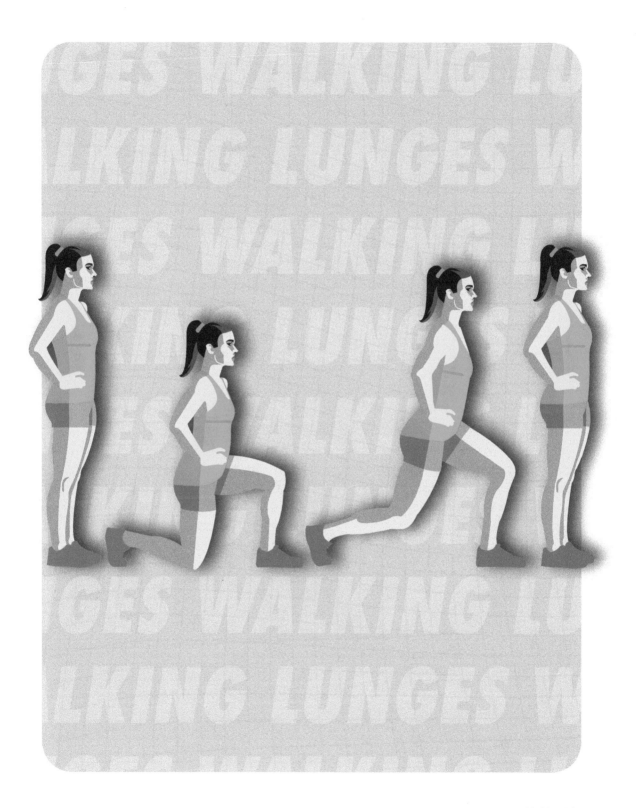

CHAIR SQUATS

I feel like this is the foundational exercise for all sports, not just running. Learning how to do this correctly is key to executing so many other movements in your daily life properly, like picking up your kids (or grandkids), shoveling snow, picking up bags of soil for the garden, grabbing clothes out of the washing machine, and on and on. Squats target your quads, hip extensors (glutes), and hamstrings without putting too much emphasis on balance.

BENEFITS: Squats build bilateral symmetry—equal strength on right and left sides—or help you work toward it. By actively, forcefully contracting these muscles, you'll be able to produce more power when accelerating on your runs, going uphill, or deploying a killer kick at the end of a race. Increased range of motion in the ankle joint is also an added bonus.

HOW TO:

1. Stand in front of a chair, with your back facing the chair, feet shoulder-width apart, knees slightly bent, arms by your sides.

2. Inhale as you engage your abs and bend your knees, pushing your hips back, as you slowly lower your bottom to touch the seat of the chair.

3. Exhale as you lift back up to starting position.

4. Do 8 to 12 reps, take a short break (1 to 2 minutes), and then repeat, doing 2 or 3 sets total.

For best results, perform this move a few times each week. Once you feel like you're completing your squats using proper form, you can add light weights to the exercise.

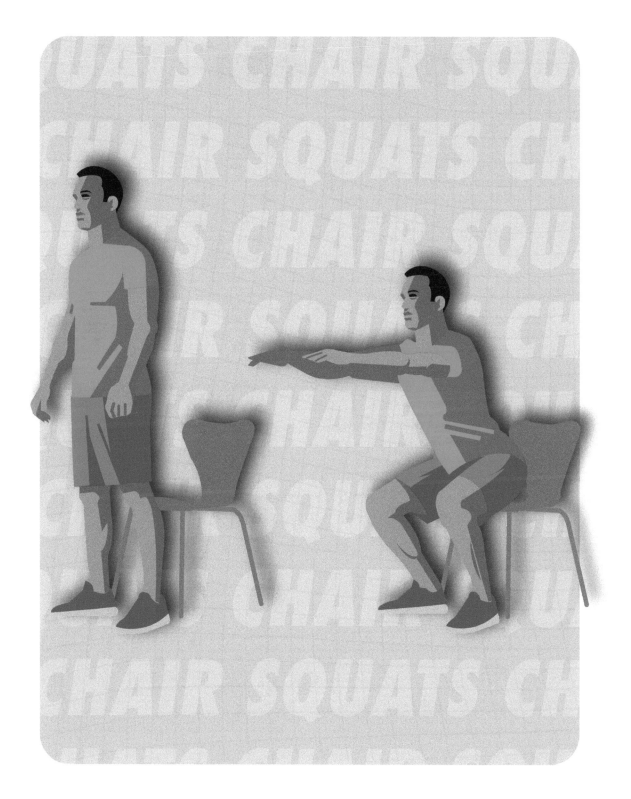

CALF RAISES

Lower leg injuries can crop up from time to time, so having toned calf muscles, along with very strong tendons and ligaments, will help keep you running strong through the most demanding of training periods. Calf raises are very easy to do and require little, if any, equipment. All you need is a short step and your own body weight.

BENEFITS: Develops strength in the gastrocnemius and soleus muscles, along with the Achilles tendon that attaches these muscles to your heel bone. Instead of waiting around to get injured and having to perform rehabilitation exercises to correct the injury, why not start "pre-hab" and get ahead of it? With the calf raise motion, you have an opportunity to stretch both your calf muscle and your Achilles, which allows for scar tissue to be broken up and promotes blood flow to heal any micro tears that may have occurred during training.

HOW TO:

1. Find a step, preferably one with a hand railing that you can use for balance.

2. Stand on the edge of the step with your feet about hip-width apart and your heels hanging off so your body weight is on your forefeet.

3. Gently lower your heels down an inch or two, until you feel a stretch and hold for 1 to 2 seconds.

4. Rise back to start and hold for 1 to 2 seconds. Repeat.

5. Do 8 to 12 reps, take a short rest, and then repeat.

For best results, perform this exercise a few times each week.

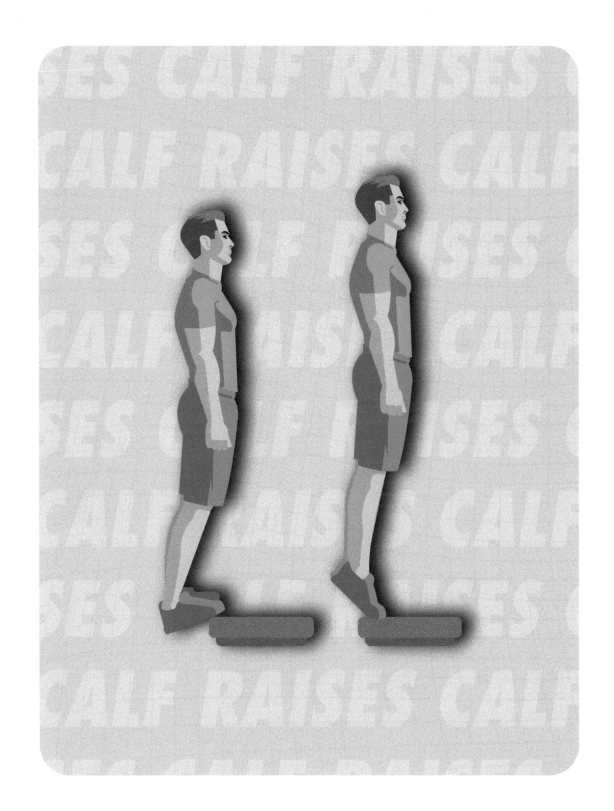

PLYOMETRIC JUMPS

Once you've nailed your traditional squats (with added weights), you're ready to perform some plyometric jumps. This type of movement is incredibly functional and helps in all aspects of our lives. Just once or twice a week can return joint fluidity back into your legs.

BENEFITS: Plyometric jumps allow you to practice high-velocity muscle contraction in the safety of a controlled setting, such as your house or a park. Plyometrics can enable a springier and speedier toe-off while running.

HOW TO:

You know how to jump, but we're going to focus on the *up* phase of this movement, really getting your feet off the ground and then landing softly, with knees slightly bent, when you come back down to reduce the impact.

1. Stand with your feet shoulder-width apart, knees slightly bent, arms by your sides.

2. Bend your knees, pushing your hips behind you in a squat, and then press into the balls of your feet and jump straight up, extending your legs and lifting feet a few inches off floor.

3. Land softly with your knees slightly bent. You can practice doing this onto a low step as well, hopping up and then stepping back down.

This exercise can be challenging at first. If it has been a while since you have jumped up and down for exercise, be sure to progress slowly to allow your body to adapt.

OPTIMIZE YOUR CADENCE

What are we trying to achieve with cadence? We should all be shooting for a rate of 160 to 180 steps per minute. The experts have deemed this frequency to be the most efficient, as we're not overstriding and we're landing softly enough to reduce our impact force and risk of injury. Regardless of whether you're running slow and easy or fast and hard, your foot strike, or cadence, should stay in that zone.

TESTING PROTOCOL

BENEFITS: A smooth stride will give you the ability to run healthy and powerfully for decades. There will be less wear and tear on your body, and you'll go through running shoes less quickly (which saves money—cha-ching!).

Time to do some math and take notes on your next treadmill session. You can also just use a GPS watch.

1. Start off at a warm-up effort and count how many steps (right and left) you take in one minute.

2. Make a note of your cadence at warm-up pace, marathon pace, long rep or tempo pace, and 5K race pace.

3. At each of these paces, your cadence should be about 5 percent greater than the previous pace, all the way up to about 180 steps per minute—your optimal target.

DOWNHILL STRIDES

When you perform strides downhill, you're literally using gravity to force your legs to turn over faster. This technique is widely used by athletes of all abilities who are seeking a way to run at 110 percent of maximum velocity. This type of running requires the body to already be warmed up, so you should always perform these after an easy run.

BENEFITS: Being forced to run at a faster pace will allow the average runner to continue to make gains in their racing performances. By running faster on a downhill grade, we are not only stressing our muscles to contract quicker so we don't fall head over heels, but we are also calling upon our nervous system to recruit our muscles to act and respond at lightning speed.

HOW TO:

1. Warm up for 30 to 60 minutes with an easy run, then do a few stretches, focusing on your hamstrings and hip flexors.

2. Find a nice, gentle-grade hill (1 to 3 percent) that's about 80 to 100 meters in length, on pavement, smooth gravel, or a dirt path.

3. Start at the top of the hill, running at an easy pace, and gradually pick up your speed and turnover rate.

4. At the end of each stride or relaxed sprint, gradually decelerate down to a walk, turn around, and walk back up to the start.

5. Do three to five reps.

CADENCE TRAINING

The backstory on this one is that when my daughter, Piper, was an infant, I would lay her on the couch or bed, grab hold of both her ankles, and put her legs through the running motion as fast as my arms would allow, saying "fast feet, fast feet" as I did it. I wanted her—and you—to know that in order to be fast, you have to think fast thoughts. Just like in the science fiction movie *The Matrix* when Morpheus is training Neo in the fight simulator and tells him, "Don't think you're fast; know you're fast." You have to believe you are fast and that you can become faster through training.

BENEFITS: By practicing being fast, you'll increase your cadence to the goal of 180 steps per minute, which should lead to better performances and fewer injuries.

HOW TO:

Again, you need to be well warmed up for this running drill, so practice this after a 30- to 60-minute easy run. This drill can be done anywhere—on grass, dirt, pavement, or down at the local track.

1. To start, use a short and quick stride, taking as many steps as fast as you can in 10 meters.

2. Walk back to recover, take a 30-second rest, and then repeat.

3. Do 5 to 10 reps. You're working on minimizing the amount of time you spend on the ground with every rep.

REST AND RECOVERY

MASSAGE

Getting regular massages may seem luxurious, but the reality is that it provides recovery from workouts and helps you stay healthy through arduous training cycles. Now, I know that a few hours of massage therapy every week is not feasible for most people, but striving to get whatever you can is beneficial, even if you're doing self-massage, like I did in college. Massaging your own legs can do wonders for recovery.

BENEFITS: Massage reduces muscle tension in your legs. The mechanics of physically pushing out the metabolic waste that has built up over the course of a few weeks as a result of hard training can help speed up the recovery process. Massage therapy can help lengthen muscle tissue back to its resting length, promoting optimal blood flow to your muscle cells, tendons, and ligaments.

DIY!

1. Put on a pair of old running shorts, grab some olive oil, and get comfortable on the floor with a towel underneath you.

2. Put a very small amount of oil on your legs, then start with long strokes on your calves and shins and gradually work your way up to your quads.

3. The hamstrings are a little hard to get to but give them a try. Spend extra time rubbing muscles that feel sore. You can also use a foam roller or ball to really get in there and work out your kinks.

Or find yourself a good massage therapist that specializes in sports massage and hold on to them with all your might. Ask around at the track, the local running store, or a physical therapy clinic—someone should be able to point you in the right direction.

LIGHT, POST-RUN STRETCHING

After a hard training session, stretching lightly can enhance your recovery process. Find a comfortable spot to sit and gently put your muscles and joints through a series of easy mobility stretches when your body is all warmed up. Dedicating a spot in your home can help motivate you to consistently stretch after a run. Think of it as your own little "pre-hab" center.

BENEFITS: Stretching promotes circulation and blood flow to the muscles that have just been put through the wringer. It also helps realign your back with better postural awareness. Take this time to decompress after your training session, reflecting on the time well spent bettering yourself and your fitness. Bottom line: Many physiological benefits occur while stretching lightly post-run.

HOW TO:

Stretching after a run can be quick; all you really need is just 5 to 10 minutes. I highly recommend *The Whartons' Stretch Book*, which illustrates the proper way to perform Active Isolate Stretching, or AIS. And if you want some visuals of the stretching routine, search YouTube videos on AIS.

Stretching is by far the best habit you can develop to keep healthy and strong for years to come.

SLEEP!

This includes naps. Sleep gives our bodies time to rebuild and recover from training and life stress, which is more and more important as we age. I advocate getting *eight* nights of sleep a week to my elite running team: The total amount of their naps during the week should add up to eight to nine hours of sleep, thus adding one extra night of sleep. Most of us don't have time to take that many naps, but try to at least sneak in one or two on the weekends, especially after your long Sunday run. I coach a few older athletes who work full-time during the week, and they just love to lay down on the couch post-run, with their eyes closed and the sun's rays shining down on them.

BENEFITS: We see a boost in human growth hormone (HGH) production after just a 30-minute nap. Strive to consistently get eight hours of sleep each and every night. Remember: We don't get stronger during a training session or workout; we tear our bodies down during the stimulus of it. It's during sleep that we rebuild our bodies, both at night while we're in REM sleep and during those shorter, day naps. Our bodies get flooded with HGH to start the reconstruction process, or "restocking our shelves," as I like to call it.

HOW TO:

Most people spend one-third of their day in bed. Get a comfortable mattress and cozy sheets. Keep in mind that you want to stay warm when you sleep, both at night or during the day, because regulating your body temperature externally allows all the energy in your body to go directly toward repairing and rebuilding. And instill calm in whatever ways you can, including getting your TV, phone, and other devices out of the bedroom. These flashing lights can play tricks on your brain, fooling it into believing it's daytime.

FOOT CONTROL

I hear a lot about hip mobility through articles or questions at coaching clinics, yet no one seems to ever talk about foot mobility and how to assess and improve it. This is also really important, especially for runners who spend a lot of time on their feet.

The major movements of our feet are generated by larger muscles in our lower legs, primarily the calf muscles (gastrocnemius and soleus), shin muscles (anterior tibialis), and those located on the sides of our leg (peroneals). If any or all of these muscle groups are tight, the big mo-tions of our feet become limited and it hinders their overall function. A great exercise that can address tightness in our shins and lateral aspect of the lower leg is **ankle circles**.

When standing, simply point one of your feet straight down so that your toes are touching the ground, then slowly circle your foot in one direction so you feel a stretch on the outside of your ankle. As you rotate, you'll feel a stretch in your shin as well. Make 8 to 10 slow circles, then switch directions and repeat.

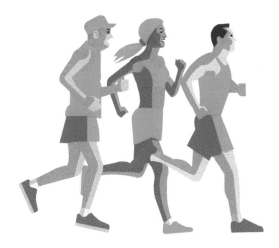

PROTEIN

GRAINS

FRUIT

GREENS

CHAPTER FOUR

INVIGORATION

NUTRITION FOR SEASONED ATHLETES

The old saying "You are what you eat" has stood the test of time for a reason; it's really that simple. Fad diets come and go, but if you eat fresh, organic vegetables and lean, grass-fed animals, then you'll look and feel healthier. And of course the inverse is true, too—if you predominantly feast on packaged products and greasy, nutrient-poor processed meats, your body will look and feel worse. What you eat is critical to procuring vitality, energy, strength, power, and our most precious commodity as runners, ENDURANCE, which is your ability to go the distance during your workouts, as well as over the years as you get older.

In this chapter, I'll be giving you some easy-to-follow advice on what to eat, based mostly on what I—and the elite athletes I coach—eat for breakfast, lunch, and dinner. This is not because I'm a registered dietician or nutrition expert (disclaimer: I'm not!), but because after years of trial and error, of training and coaching (and reading about nutrition, training and coaching!), I honestly know what helps optimize performance and why. I've seen small dietary changes totally transform an athlete's performance.

Our main focus in this chapter will be identifying nutrient-dense foods, or foods that contain a large quantity of nutrients, like essential vitamins, minerals, antioxidants, unsaturated fats, and fiber, but that yield a low number of calories that will help fuel your workouts—and your busy life. We'll also talk about the much-heralded superfoods, like kale, spinach, broccoli, quinoa, fish, and the health benefits they provide to runners in particular.

Last, but not least, we'll discuss the timing of meals and snacks and how this can affect your performance. Learning when it is best to consume calories and nutrients is critical as a runner. Certain foods are better to consume right before you work out, while others are best saved for right after, or even during. I know, if you're reading this book, it's likely that you've been running for a long time and you already have a sense of what works for you. However, as we age, nutrition and self-assessment just get more and more important. I'll help you look at your habits with fresh eyes and prepare to optimize and protect your performance for the years to come.

EATING FOR POWER AND ENDURANCE

I met coach Joe Vigil in my early 20s. Since then, we have shared many cups of coffee and stories about runners and training. During one of our notorious coffeehouse "save the world" discussions, he said something that I'll never forget. Joe looked at me and said, "Andrew, you're only as good as you want to be." I have applied this quote, motto, and philosophy to many aspects of my life. When my motivation is low and other distractions come to the forefront, I tell myself, "You're only as good as you want to be. How good do I want to be? How much time and energy is required of me to complete this task, this workout, this meal, to be as good as I want to be?" When I ask myself those questions, the answer, inevitably, is always that whatever I'm putting in is worth it in order to reach my goals.

I encourage you to apply this attitude to your diet and nutritional plan, too. You're only as good or as healthy as you want to be. If you're eating only processed foods or ordering take-out all the time and drinking too much alcohol, then you're telling yourself and your body that you don't really want to be that good at what you're doing. And I know that's not true. Just by picking up this book, you're saying that you're better than that. You're trying to learn something, trying to improve the longevity of your running . . . and your life in general.

A runner who wants to be good, who wants to run healthy and strong for decades to come, will make the changes needed to do so. You'll seek out nutrient-dense, antioxidant-rich foods that offer more bang for your buck. These foods will boost your health, your energy, and your performance now and help diminish the wear and tear of time on your body. And when you feel better overall, then you'll feel better out on the road or trail. I promise.

RECONSIDER YOUR DIET

When I think of the word "diet," I think of fads and trendy eating habits that promise quick results. But the reality is, it's all about choosing a healthier lifestyle and emulating the way some people have approached food for hundreds of years. Let's look at the Mediterranean diet, for example. People from the Mediterranean (Crete, Greece, and Southern Italy) are typically healthier, thinner, and live longer than people from other areas around the world. Their culture—how they ate and lived—became of interest to US researchers back in the 1960s when heart disease was on the rise here and they were looking for ways to reverse the trend.

Not only does a Mediterranean lifestyle promote the consumption of whole grains, fish, olives, nuts (all of which contain "good" fats), vegetables, fruits, and very little high-fat meats, it also emphasizes dining with family and friends, sourcing locally, and being active in your daily routine.

I've experienced firsthand the health benefits that are often associated with the Mediterranean diet. Back in 2004, I spent three weeks on the island of Crete, as it was home to the United States Olympic Track and Field Team in their preparation for the Athens Summer Olympics. At our resort, we ate locally grown fruits and vegetables, olive oil, fish, and lean meat that was slaughtered within hours of being served. Everything we consumed was sourced within a five-mile radius—so it was as fresh as possible. Looking back on that time, I honestly think I have never been healthier. Our US Olympic Team did fairly well at those Games, too, come to think of it. Coincidence? I think not.

But people across the Mediterranean aren't the only ones doing it right. National Geographic Fellow (and *New York Times* best-selling author) Dan Buettner discovered that people living in seven identified "Blue Zones" around the world live longer than everyone else due to factors such as diet, exercise, interpersonal relationships, and overall lifestyle choices.

Further, the latest research from the field of epigenetics finds that, while genes play a role in longevity, diet and lifestyle may be bigger influences, turning off positive and negative gene expressions that dramatically affect how we age. Therefore, it's helpful to study the cultures that produce healthy older adults and the highest numbers of centenarians—the Blue Zones.

What are the folks in these magically healthy Blue Zones eating, you ask? Here's a brief breakdown of their optimized existence:

» Ninety-five percent of their food items are plant-based.

» They stop eating when 80 percent full.

» They eat ½ cup of beans daily.

» The biggest meal is breakfast; the smallest is dinner.

» Many snack on a handful of nuts daily.

» They cook a majority of their meals at home.

What to eat . . .

» Beans

» Greens, like spinach, kale, chards, beet tops, fennel tops, collards

» Sweet potatoes

» Nuts

» Extra-virgin olive oil

» Oats (slow-cooked or Irish steel-cut)

» Barley

» Fruit

» Green or herbal tea

» Turmeric (spice or tea)

» Fish

» Pastured, organic meats

» Organic, nonhomogenized dairy

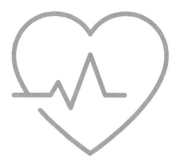

FOODS TO INCLUDE AND FOODS TO AVOID

FOODS TO INCLUDE IN YOUR DIET	WHY?
Whole grains	Another food that helps reduce cholesterol and boost the satiated, or full/satisfied, feeling you get when you eat. Consume these either before or after a run and be sure to add a protein (yogurt or milk) to repair tissue damage.
Citrus fruit, like oranges, grapefruit, kiwi, and mangos	These give you an antioxidant boost of vitamin C, a nutrient that helps reduce muscle damage while training and simultaneously amps up your immune system.
Dark, leafy greens	Greens, like iron-rich spinach, are great for your red blood cells. They're also a good source of vitamin A, K, B_2, and C, and are essential for maintaining bone health. A bonus benefit: They contain chlorophyll, which has special cancer-fighting properties.
Nuts	A great source of vitamin E, nuts have been shown to lower cholesterol levels and protect against certain cancers. Eat a handful of nuts several times per week as a snack or sprinkle them on top of a salad.
Eggs (3 to 5 per week)	The most complete protein available to us, one egg can account for about 10 percent of your daily protein requirements. The yolk contains vitamins A, D, E, B_{12}, and K, along with folate and omega-3 fatty acids.
Sweet potatoes or yams	These root veggies provide a lot of dietary fiber and contain many vitamins and minerals such as iron, calcium, selenium, vitamin B, and vitamin C. Fun fact: Usain Bolt claims the real secret to his sprinting success is the yams his mother cooked when he was growing up.

FOODS TO INCLUDE AND FOODS TO AVOID

FOODS TO EXCLUDE IN YOUR DIET	WHY?
Margarine	This fake butter is processed in a lab, high in trans fats, and contains omega-6 fats (which promote inflammation), emulsifiers, additives, colorings, and artificial flavors.
Dried and canned fruits	These are very high in concentrated sugars that can promote weight gain and do little to curb hunger. You're always better off going fresh.
Bacon	It contains a high amount of saturated fat, which is linked to coronary artery disease. Most cuts of packaged bacon also contain preservatives that have been linked to certain cancers.
Sugary cereals and granola bars	Minerals and vitamins are stripped from refined grains during processing. Sugar has been found to feed cancer cells and contribute to arthritis, too.
Condiments, like ketchup and mustard	Unless homemade, these are mostly a combination of sugar and chemicals.
"Healthy" frozen meals	The goal of these types of meals is to control portion size and limit calories. However, they're usually lacking in nutrients and high in sodium. They're also less satisfying than a freshly prepared meal.

What to avoid . . .

» Large servings of meat (at most, consume twice a week and just a couple of ounces is plenty)

» Processed dairy daily (limit to a few small servings two to three times a week)

» Eggs (at most, consume three eggs a week)

» Sugar (limit as much as possible)

» Heavily processed flours and "de-natured" common foods

Again, how people in the Blue Zones eat is only one aspect of why they continue to thrive over time. Also working in their favor is the priority placed on cooking with family and friends, exercising, gardening, staying both mentally and physically active, consuming low amounts of alcohol, and living with purpose, or giving back to their communities and society.

CALORIC NEEDS OF RUNNERS

With so many people counting calories while dieting over the years, the fact that calories equal energy often gets lost in translation. So as a runner, in particular, getting enough—though not too many—calories is essential. But figuring out how many calories you need every day (i.e., your daily caloric intake) can be tricky. There are many factors at play, including your gender, age, weight, height, and how many miles you're running per day.

Sports nutritionist Trevor Bedding recommends using the following formula to determine your caloric intake:

Step 1: Calculate your resting metabolic rate (RMR).

» If you are female, age 31 to 60 years:
(Body weight in kg x 8.7) + 829

» If you are male, age 31 to 60 years:
(Body weight in kg x 11.6) + 879

Step 2: Based on your daily physical activity, calculate your daily energy expenditure. Multiply your RMR by the following measure:

» If you do very little/no exercise x 1.4

» If you are moderately active x 1.7

» If you are very active x 2.0

Step 3: Calculate how many calories you burn each week through running (an approximate guide will be 100 calories/mile*). Divide this by seven to find your daily average.

Step 4: Add the figures obtained from steps 2 and 3 to find your maintenance intake. If you eat this number of calories per day, based on your current training regime, you will stay at the same weight.

Step 5: Reduce your caloric intake by 15 percent if you wish to lose weight. Multiply your maintenance calories by 0.85 percent to give you a new caloric total.

Here is an example for a 45-year-old male who weighs 165 pounds (75kg), is very active, and runs 40 miles per week.

Step 1: 75 kg x 11.6 = 870 + 879 = 1,749

Step 2: 1,749 x 2 = 3,498

Step 3: 40 miles per week x 100* = 4,000 ÷ 7 = 571 calories burned each day from running.

Step 4: Add 3,498 calories to 571 calories and we get 4,069 calories needed if this person wants to maintain their current body weight from week to week. If they want to lose weight, slice off 15 percent of calories needed to go into caloric deficiency for weight loss. That formula would be 4,069 x 0.85 or 15 percent = 3,458 calories.

*On average, we burn 100 to 125 calories per mile run, depending on our size and pace (the smaller we are and the slower we run, the fewer calories we burn).

NUTRIENT ALLIES

In order to function well or perform optimally at any age, our bodies need to be fueled properly. We require nutrients, minerals, vitamins, and calories provided by carbohydrates, proteins, and fats to provide energy and sustenance.

Our tissues are constantly being broken down and then remolded. We have to seek out well-engineered and high-quality building blocks (i.e., nutrient-dense foods) throughout this process in order to promote growth to our infrastructure and framework.

The building blocks you need most as a runner are carbs, proteins, and fats. Whoever labeled any of these components as "bad" was not logging miles regularly, that's for sure. All three have a time, a place, and a purpose, and all three come in a variety of forms.

Both simple and complex carbohydrates are needed at certain times of the day. When our elite Mammoth Track Club athletes are "in season," I offer some pretty basic nutritional advice for them: Limit sugars (simple carbohydrates) outside of the training session or workout. Consuming sugars—in the form of sports drinks or gels—during training is advocated by just about every sports nutritionist and endurance sports scientist out there. Coach Vigil always used to say, "Fat burns in a carbohydrate flame."

As you probably know, marathon runners derive the lion's share of their energy demands while running from the fat or adipose they carry on their bodies. Fat is the most efficient fuel source for low-intensity running, or aerobically based endurance activity, due to its caloric density. But one can best harness the energy from fat by priming their system with simple carbs.

Complex carbohydrates can help restock the stored energy in glycogen, our muscle cells. When we start moving and contracting muscle tissue, we need energy and this is where the stored glycogen comes into play, acting as a source of energy for repetitive muscle contractions.

Believe it or not, fat is a hugely important component in your diet, too. Not only do we store fat to use as energy later, we need it to rebuild and repair tissues. Cell membranes have a fatty acid derivative and neurons have a sheath around the axon that's made of fat for conductivity. The cholesterol that sits on top of our skin converts the sun's rays to vitamin D, and even that comes from the fats we eat.

Protein also supplies our muscles with energy, but only after carbohydrates and fats have been called upon first; usually not until after at least 90 minutes of exercise. We mainly use them for recovery from the destructive aftermath of exercise. Consuming good sources of protein should be a priority in the lives of everyone, especially runners. Due to the near infinite amount of sport science research out there on the "athlete diet," it is my opinion that a small amount of meat goes a long way when it comes to repairing tissues of the aging runner. Also, a combination of whole grains, such as quinoa, kamut, wild rice, millet, and oats, and protein goes a long way in aiding muscle recovery.

Vitamin C plays a very important role in rebuilding various body tissues in the following ways:

» Produces some neurotransmitters.

» Boosts collagen, which provides strength in many tissues of the body and helps maintain healthy skin.

» Helps metabolize proteins.

- » Has antiaging attributes.

- » Anti-inflammatory properties assist in wound and infection healing.

- » The best food source of vitamin C is citrus fruits, like oranges and grapefruit, as well as broccoli, green and red peppers, spinach, and cabbage.

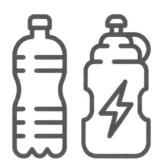

BLOOD SUGAR AWARENESS

As you know, a lot of things change as we get older—some are more noticeable than others. And even though we can't physically see it happening, our organs function a little differently with each passing year. Our pancreas, an organ with endocrine function nestled deep in our abdomen, helps convert the food we eat into energy that's then used by our muscles and other organs. As we age, the function of this organ tends to diminish, leading to an increase of unwanted blood sugar, and possibly the development of diabetes. But the good news is that your blood sugar can be regulated in part with consistent, daily running and a nutrient-dense, well-balanced diet, leading to steady glucose levels in the blood and better brain, liver, and kidney function.

As runners, we are prone to spikes in our blood sugar levels, with activities like carbo-loading before a big race or long training run. And while there is definitely a time and place for this type of eating, your goal should be to try and maintain a steady blood sugar level most of the time. Also, you should prep your body for these occasional spikes by incorporating carbo-loading into your training. At least three to five times during a training cycle or half marathon/marathon build-up, eat a similar meal or meals to what you would eat pre-race in the hours/days leading up to an important training run. You can also practice this before a shorter, less important race that's built into your schedule.

These meals should contain complex carbohydrates, such as whole grain pastas and breads, as well as potatoes, rice, and other grains. The goal is not to stuff yourself; overeating the night before a race could lead to an unwanted bathroom break when you least expect it the following morning. Just aim to fill yourself to about 80 percent capacity.

Unfortunately, our risk of developing diabetes increases as we age, but running can help reduce that risk (phew!). In general, logging regular miles helps lower your blood sugar by increasing sensitivity to insulin, thereby increasing your body's ability to use glycogen to fuel your muscles and organs.

Follow this "recipe" to maintain a healthy blood sugar level:

1. Before exercise, eat a meal rich in complex carbohydrates (toast, oatmeal, or rice).

2. Allow 60 to 90 minutes for digestion before starting a run.

3. If the run is over one hour in length, consider taking a sports drink containing carbohydrates and electrolytes with you and sip it every 15 to 20 minutes.

4. After your training run (within about 30 to 45 minutes), eat a meal rich in carbohydrates, fats, and proteins. This helps restock your carbohydrate stores for the next training session.

5. Avoid simple sugar consumption during the rest of the day!

FRENEMIES: SUGAR, CAFFEINE, AND ALCOHOL

SUGAR

Genetically, we are predisposed to crave simple sugars for quick energy. It's hard to stay disciplined, even if you know you shouldn't be consuming sugar all the time, since we live in a world where candy, sweets, and other sugary treats are pretty much at our disposal at all times. Having bite-size refined sugars readily available makes it all the more difficult to choose foods that help us live a long and healthy life. When you eat sweet treats, you are really seeking immediate gratification versus continuing along a path of achieving a long and disease-free life. I honestly hate Halloween and nearly every other holiday out there that praises the consumption of sugar for this very reason.

When and How to Consume Products with Sugar

I suggest the runners I coach consume three to five ounces of a fluid carbohydrate replacement (sports) drink every 20 to 30 minutes while they're exercising. This could be during a track session or a slow, easy long run. During this time, simple sugars are okay in my book. Outside of this, however, refined simple sugars should be avoided. I know that's not totally realistic, but that's the strategy for optimal performance and health benefits.

CAFFEINE

Recent studies have shown that a particular gene determines the rate at which you metabolize caffeine—and it varies for everyone. The only way to find out if you metabolize caffeine rapidly or slowly is to take a genetic test, which I realize most of us are not going to do anytime soon. But the reality is that for slow metabolizers, caffeine may build up in their systems and upset their stomachs, disrupt their sleep patterns, or even lead to anxiety.

Caffeine is a stimulant that's found in coffee, green and black teas, soda, energy drinks, and chocolate. It acts upon and heightens the sensitivity of your central nervous system. One single eight-ounce cup of coffee contains about 95mg of caffeine. But the amount of caffeine in various coffee drinks can range from about zero to over 500mg! It depends on how the drink is processed and packaged with other ingredients.

Deena's never been tested, but I suspect my wife possesses the fast-burning caffeine gene, whereas I know for sure that I have the slow-processing one. I limit my coffee and caffeine intake to just one cup a day, usually about 90 minutes before my morning run. Once I get back from my run, I know that I've metabolized the caffeine consumed, along with the bagel or oatmeal I ate earlier that morning. This allows me to go through the day without any of the ups or downs that are often caused by consuming copious amounts of coffee whenever I feel like it.

When I drink regular coffee in the afternoon, I am met with some challenges. I feel jittery, my stomach can turn queasy or gaseous, and I always have a slight to major disruption in my nocturnal sleep patterns as a result. If I'm in a social situation at the coffee shop and it's between 2 p.m. and 4 p.m., I may order decaf, but even then, the acid in the coffee can still have an ill effect on my stomach. If these symptoms sound all too familiar to you, then you probably possess the slow-metabolism gene, too. So be warned! Take it easy on the coffee, teas, and chocolate. You'll feel—and run—better for it.

When and How to Consume Products with Caffeine

Many runners utilize the performance benefits of this stimulant. So much so, in fact, that it was on the global banned performance-enhancing substance list (in very high quantities) up until 2003. Coffee can get your intestines and central nervous system going in the morning. It also helps to mobilize free fatty acids for enhanced energy production. From your gut to the bloodstream, caffeine is rapidly absorbed and will peak around 90 minutes later, so if you're looking for a little boost during your workout, plan accordingly. Otherwise, I would recommend limiting coffee to about one cup day, if possible.

ALCOHOL

I have found you can find something online to support just about any position you choose to support your bias or habits. Countless articles tout the benefits of having one glass of wine a night, from lowering your cholesterol levels and blood pressure, to making your bones more robust, to injecting your diet with antioxidants and vitamins.

In the running industry, both my wife and I are known for being wine connoisseurs. We love to bring the gift of wine from our favorite regions to race directors and elite athlete coordinators, sharing our passion for the fermented grapes. We've gone so far as to center our running camps in Mammoth Lakes around a running and wine experience. In fact, the night before the Olympic Marathon in 2004, Deena and I enjoyed a glass of wine with dinner, celebrating all the hard work that got her to that point of her career.

I've personally found that consuming one alcoholic drink will likely have little to no effect on my racing or training performance, but several drinks most definitely will! Indulging in too much in wine or beer can and will have a negative effect on your performance the next morning, whether it's a race or a workout. This is mainly due to dehydration, since alcohol is a diuretic. Additionally, it diminishes the uptake of glucose and amino acids of your muscles, not to mention the fact that consuming alcohol the night before a workout or race may adversely affect your body's temperature regulation and disrupt your sleep.

When I was in high school, my cross-country running coach told each of us on the team that alcohol was bad for our running, not to mention that it was illegal to consume it at our age. He always said that it destroyed the aerobic enzymes that we worked so hard to create during intense training sessions. I don't know that there's evidence to prove that's true, but I do know plenty of elite runners who abstain from alcohol for various reasons. I think you have to listen to your body and make your own choices, but know that too much of anything can definitely have negative consequences on your life and your running.

When and How to Consume Products with Alcohol

I do agree that "a glass of wine has healthy benefits that keep the doctor away." Wine, over other alcoholic beverages, does possess minerals, vitamins, and antioxidants. Plus, there are true mental health benefits to sitting around with family and friends enjoying a glass of wine here and there. Consume your wine on the harder workout days. You'll need to exercise some discipline on the evenings before a race or a hard workout, and remember, you will most likely suffer the consequences of having too good of a time, especially as you get older.

WHEN AND WHY TO SUPPLEMENT

Eating well and getting vital nutrients becomes increasingly important as we age. There is simply a smaller margin for error with our nutritional balance, due to the risk of breaking bones and becoming susceptible to diseases and illnesses. But as you know, getting 100 percent of vitamins and minerals from our diet becomes increasingly difficult, and our body's ability to absorb nutrients can diminish as we age. That's where supplements come in.

As with any big behavioral change to your health or nutrition routine, you should discuss your supplementation needs with your doctors first. They can perform a thorough blood panel to reveal potential deficiencies in certain vitamins and minerals. Don't just go shopping at the health food store and purchase $200 worth of supplements you think you might need. Typically, any deficiencies found can be addressed fairly quickly, and retesting in three to four months can reveal whether the supplements you're taking are actually helping to restore mineral and vitamin levels back to their "normal" ranges.

One of the more common deficiencies found is in vitamin D. Maintaining a normal level of vitamin D is extraordinarily important because, among other benefits, it has been found to improve our immune function, aid in recovery from tough workouts, and boost athletic performance in elite runners, which is why vitamin D is usually consumed in large quantities by these athletes. Unlike a lot of other vitamins, D can be easily absorbed in two different ways: (1) through the consumption of green leafy vegetables, fish, and dairy products, and (2) sun exposure. When sunlight hits our skin, cholesterol molecules produced in the dermis synthesize the UVB rays into vitamin D to be absorbed into the bloodstream. So make sure you're getting enough sunlight during the day. I tell my athletes to only wash their faces and stinky parts (in that order!) in the shower with soap, as I want them to keep the cholesterol molecules in their skin on their arms, legs, and abdomen.

Another important element to watch is ferritin, which your body uses to transport oxygen (via hemoglobin). A low level of ferritin is an indicator for anemia, which is, unfortunately, common among runners. The more you run and train, the more susceptible you are to displaying signs of anemia (extreme fatigue, pale skin, cold hands and feet, and craving shaved ice).

Again, rather than self-diagnosing and trying to create a magical mix of supplements for yourself, talk to your doctor and learn what deficiencies you may have that actually need to be addressed.

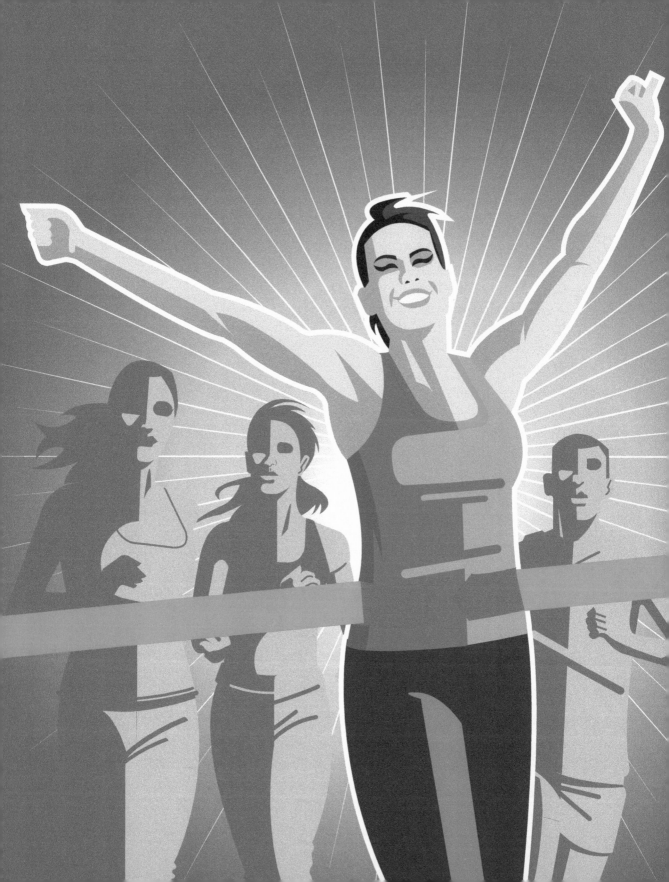

CHAPTER FIVE

REINVENTION

EMOTIONAL RESILIENCE AND ADAPTABILITY

We've already spent a lot of time discussing the physical challenges and limitations runners face as they get older. But that's really only half of it—there's a whole other side of the equation that needs to be addressed and explored, too. What happens to us mentally, emotionally, and spiritually over time affects how we live and run. You have to train both your mind *and* your body, period. If you're not mentally strong, then chances are you're not going to feel physically strong or perform your best out on the road. In this chapter, we'll discuss the mental and emotional benefits of running at any age, how you can boost those throughout the decades, and find an honest answer to that "Why do you run?" question you get asked so often.

Running charges me physically, emotionally, and socially. It's an activity that can keep us connected to friends and our fitness levels up, no matter how old (or slow!) we get. Taking time to consider what running does for you, personally, is important. Is it your reason for getting up in the morning— seeing the sunrise as you run with a friend, followed by coffee? Or are you motivated by more external forces, like watching your favorite TV show while you log miles on the treadmill? Why you run and how it makes you feel as a result will likely help determine whether you stick with it as you get older and the miles get harder. One would hope that we'd all become more dedicated to the process, staying fitter and healthier than ever before, but you just never know. These are individual questions that only you can answer, but we can—and should— explore them together.

ENJOYING EACH STEP

We all have different reasons to run and different goals we're trying to reach, and they're changing constantly. My current goal, at 42, for example, is to run a mile as fast as I did when I was 14 (4:50) during my very first track season. This is a challenging but doable feat—as long as I put in the work each day. Sure, a decade ago my goals and schedule looked very different, but it's something worth striving for; we all need something to chase to drive us further and farther.

My friend Rick Wood is another example. I've known Rick, a 68-year-old attorney, former mayor, and avid runner who still logs 50 to 60 hours a week at his law practice, for about 13 years. He's the guy up at 4 a.m. running around in the dark or watching political news shows on the treadmill. Although he did run a couple of cross-country seasons in high school and a couple of miles per day throughout his 30s and 40s, he really didn't start running competitively until he was 55. He has run about 10 half and full marathons since.

He took up running because he noticed that those in his social circle were looking old, out of shape, and unhealthy. Since he wanted no part of that downward spiral, he hired me to coach him. I set up his weekly training plan, helped lay out a racing calendar, and developed race strategies that would carry him to the number one spot in his age group. Rick really likes to win—in the courtroom and on the racecourse—and running has become a big part of his identity.

In addition to winning and beating his own personal bests in every distance possible, Rick also has a simple goal of maintaining a healthy lifestyle and a slim waistline. He is the same weight and has the same 29-inch waistline today as he did in high school.

Whatever your goals are, they have to be achievable and motivational. They should both push you and serve you at the same time. People are constantly seeking the fountain of youth and will go to extreme lengths to find it, with things like fancy creams and expensive procedures. Recognize that running can play a very natural part in maintaining youth. We are changing, our bodies are changing, and we need to deal with it the best we can—one mile at a time.

RUN TO FIGHT AILMENTS

Running is the closest thing we have to a magic bullet or an age-defying miracle pill. Regularly engaging in this activity can help fight off many common ailments that are simply a result of daily wear and tear on our bodies. But there are some physical changes that are simply inevitable as we get older.

So the question is, how do we maintain a healthy and happy perspective while adapting to our ever-changing bodies? One simple solution is to surround yourself with others who support and motivate you through the miles. Getting older is an experience we can all relate to (some obviously more than others right now, but they'll have their turn, too—don't worry!), so you shouldn't ever feel like you have to go at it alone. Sharing the miles and the reps with like-minded people and striving toward a goal with a team is both fun and inspiring. It also becomes a built-in support system, which is helpful at all ages, but especially as we grow older. Knowing that you have a crew (and possibly a coach, like me) cheering for you both on and off the track will do wonders for your psyche, your energy, and your mood.

We were all born to run. We were also born to run with others—like hunting in a pack, finding strength in numbers, that whole bit. Have you ever felt the synergy that forms from working out with others? Maybe you've experienced this in a race. Each person feeds off the energy of the other runners, not to mention the actual wind-drafting effect you get while running with the pack. Having teammates lifts us up, whether it's intentional or not.

WHY YOU SHOULD STILL RUN AS YOU AGE

As I mentioned earlier in the book, I know how hard it can be to feel yourself slow down over the years, even if you know it's only natural. There's a reason that Boston Marathon–qualifying times tick up with every age group. But if you're competitive, driven, and goal-oriented (hi, I see you!), then staying positive while your speed starts declining can be tough. I think it's important to remember that your goal should always be to be your best self. And there are ways to optimize your time, money, and energy to make the most of what you've got at any age. This book is a good starting point, and I'm here to help.

In general, our muscles don't respond like they used to and it takes longer to recover from workouts and races. These inevitable changes can be hard to get our heads around. I've chatted with older athletes plenty of times and they all same the same thing: "I still feel like I'm in my 30s and 40s, but my times and training have gradually been slipping." Again, surround yourself with others who understand, because you're not alone.

It's helpful to try to keep things in perspective and stay lighthearted with your approach. I've been competing in running events since I was a 14-year-old high school freshman. I estimate that I've toed the starting line of almost 300 races in the last 30 years. I remember the races in those early years being incredibly stressful—I would get so nervous before each race to the point of wanting to throw-up about 20 minutes before the starting gun. Then in college, something shifted: I became more focused, a bit more relaxed, and performed better each year. Fast forward just a few years, and now I don't get nervous at all before a race. I'm super-relaxed and confident, which is a feeling that I believe can only develop over time, and it allows me to perform my best. I know there is less on the line and less pressure; that it's all for *me* these days. And there is something so rewarding and refreshing about knowing that you're not doing it for points or for your teammates; you're just doing it for yourself. It's harder to find those things as we get older, and it feels really good when we do.

I highly recommend taking some of the pressure off yourself and cutting back on the all-too-common stress and anxiety before a race. I chat with others before races and workouts to find out how they're doing, what their expectations for the race are, how their training went leading up to the race—just chit-chat. Believe it or not, focusing on others can help calm you down, get out of your own head, and allow you to thrive when it's actually go-time.

The elite athletes I coach sometimes have problems finding time to connect with friends and family outside of running (understandably so!). They get so caught up in the whole eat/sleep/run/recover routine that making plans for extra activities simply doesn't happen. But finding a way to connect with people outside of your running circle is healthy and encouraged. Join a new group, start a new hobby, find people who share similar outside interests, or catch up with old friends whom you haven't

seen in a while. You'll benefit so much from being more balanced, I promise.

I've recently been noticing a lot of wine bars offering weekly painting classes. These "paint and sips" are a great way to get out, be social, and meet other people from different backgrounds with similar interests.

Another feel-good way to meet new people (if you're looking for ideas, anyway) is to volunteer. Volunteers are needed all the time! Our Mammoth Track Club organization produces a few small running events each year, and we are always looking for volunteers to help out. It often ends up being the same 12 or so volunteers signing up each time, so they really get to know each other—and the runners—over the course of the season.

ACCEPT YOURSELF

As runners, we can be very hard on ourselves. In team sports, we rely on teammates to score a goal or make a basket with the assistance of others. But in running, ultimately, it's just us out there, alone with our thoughts. If you don't perform as well as you had hoped, then the person you're most likely to turn on is yourself. This is a slippery slope, and it doesn't lead to any good results in the end. My advice: Take it easy on yourself. The sport (and everything else, really) will be much more enjoyable if you can have some self-compassion and accept who you are and your current fitness level. After all, we're runners because we choose to be, not because we have to be—so be proud of whatever strides you make and remember to keep it fun out there.

Self-acceptance is probably the best gift we can give ourselves as we get older. Our younger selves may have collected awards, gotten promotions, or snagged PRs (personal records) at every race, but it becomes more difficult to achieve those types of wins regularly as we age. However, there are other wins. It's all about putting things in perspective and giving yourself credit where credit's due. Those small day-to-day victories will become increasingly important.

Once a competitor, always a competitor; throughout our adult lives and into our senior years, our competitiveness doesn't just go away. It simply rears its head in other ways. You compete against yourself more, you compete in other arenas, and you find ways to turn things into competitions that will drive your friends and family members bananas. That competitiveness needs to be cultivated and directed in order for us to continue on with purpose and satisfaction. With that said, we need to recalibrate and redefine what our personal bests are. I suggest keeping records of age-group personal best times or records. Or look at age-graded performance calculators to compare your times over your entire running career. By looking at performances through this lens, you'll realize that your slower times may not really be as slow as you think, comparatively speaking.

RUNNER'S HIGH AND CHEMISTRY CHANGES

The "runner's high" is real. If you've been running for a while, then you know this to be true. It is a feeling that only runners can understand and is one of the many reasons we choose to continue logging miles well past our prime. But what exactly is the runner's high? German researchers have recently said the euphoric feeling we experience during running is generated by the release of endorphins or opiates into the brain (prefrontal and limbic regions). This chemical is engineered similarly to morphine in how it buffers pain sensations. Some experts have said the origin of this physiological response to aerobic exercise likely stems from when our ancestors had to chase down dinner millions of years ago. *Persistence hunting*, the act of wearing down your prey, could have lasted as long as a few hours.

Unfortunately, it can sometimes be challenging to capture this high as we get older. This could be due to several different factors, including a cascading effect all around, reduced blood flow in the body, reduced sensitivity to the endorphins being released, having a diet that lacks the nutrients possible to form endorphins with the same potency as decades ago, and the list can go on and on. But don't worry—there's still hope for us.

Going back to the whole concept of running down our prey millions of years ago... In observing my own elite track team, athletes have the tendency to perform better in workouts when they're running in a pack of others with similar physical capabilities. I can only speculate that there's an increase in endorphin production when running together. If you don't have a group to train with every day, then grab your phone (or your Sony Walkman, depending on how old you actually are—ha!), throw on your headphones and listen to some groovy tunes while you run.

In October 2019, Eliud Kipchoge broke the two-hour barrier for the marathon distance in Vienna, Austria. This was an elaborate, staged event set up strategically for one man to crack the mythical barrier. Much hype surrounded the live event in which Kipchoge reportedly received upward of $50 million for his unearthly performance. The organizers of the event wanted a live audience, a few thousand spectators screaming their heads off as he passed by on the circuit course. In Kipchoge's previous attempt at the barrier, which took place two years prior and at a secluded Formula 1 racecourse in Italy, there were no spectators or fans present to cheer on their hero.

During this record-breaking event, pace-making duties were shared by a stable of 15 highly trained men who would cycle through every 5K to keep the pace moving and shelter Kipchoge from any wind drag. What I thought was interesting, in addition to the five pacemakers in front of him, was the fact that he had two pacemakers behind him, off each shoulder a bit, where he could only sense them and maybe, on occasion, see them in his peripheral vision. I pondered the reasoning of their presence. What I came up with was that they served the purpose of keeping him mentally engaged, as if they were a threat of beating him to the finish line. I believe the formation of pacemakers was to achieve a subconscious hormonal response to keep him pressing for the finish line. Engineered endorphin exploitation, achieved!

My two takeaways from the extreme example above are that you should train in groups and listen to music to get the feel-good mojo for endurance running. The ultimate goal for all of us is to derive joy from this sport through the decades. Yeah sure, running fast times and landing yourself on the podium at a local 10K is great and all, but having a deeper purpose for why you're training every day, stretching, foam rolling, precisely timing your meals, and so on... will keep you going longer.

Having a long-range outlook is important when we're talking about sustaining a healthy lifestyle. Some people go on diets that put them into calorie deficit, but that's not sustainable. They are not changing their habits; they're looking for a quick fix to lose unwanted pounds. It's those of us who have developed sound, healthy habits over the decades that will keep running strong for many years to come.

HOW TO BUILD A BETTER MORNING ROUTINE

Let's talk about your habits for a minute. We'll start by looking at our morning routines, because this is when most of us perform our training.

Start fresh: In order to have a good run every morning, you need to be well hydrated. I make it a habit to drink eight to ten ounces of water as soon as I wake up, with no exceptions. This helps lube up my muscles and tendons, not to mention the intestines! This glass of water is followed closely by a couple of pieces of toast and a cup of coffee.

Get your run in as early as possible: If you want to run by 7 a.m., then you probably need to get up by 6 a.m., at the latest, so you can get dressed, have something healthy to eat, and use the bathroom before you hit the road.

Ease into it: Always start off slowly with a walk to loosen up, then progress to a jog. A slow progression will help reduce the wear and tear on your body and make the run feel better.

Do a post-run stretch: Leave enough time in your busy morning routine for a good stretch after your run and commit to it every single session. Remember, life takes effort in order to achieve something great. Even just five minutes can make a big difference.

Refuel: Always replenish your body after a tough training session. The first thing I consume after a run is a nourishing, powder-based green drink, followed by a nutrient-packed brunch, like a vegetable-egg scramble.

All of these habits are things you can easily incorporate into your lifestyle and will help you run happier and longer.

UNDERSTANDING THE ROLE OF HORMONES

While lifestyle and behavioral changes can impact how we feel physically and emotionally, it's also directly connected to what's going on inside our bodies, with our hormones. The endocrine system is responsible for the production of all of the natural chemicals floating around in your body, such as endorphins, which we've already discussed, as well as dopamine and testosterone.

Hormone fluctuations are an inevitable part of the aging process, and while they do affect how we run and feel, there's no need to try modifying them. I'm an advocate for a clean sport—always have been, always will be. I have seen what hard work, dedication, and training at high altitudes in the Sierra Nevada mountains of California can do for world-class runners. Athletes can achieve great things without the use of performance-enhancing drugs, like human growth hormone, testosterone, and erythropoietin (EPO).

There's a culture of aging athletes who have pursued unethical methods of achieving success. They justify such cheating in these terms: They're not robbing anyone of prize money in their age category or denying a clean competitor a spot on an Olympic team. The scary thing about going down such a road is the unpredictable health risks associated with adding hormones to your body when you really don't need them. Repeat after me: It's just NOT WORTH IT. Remember, your goal is to be the best version of yourself possible.

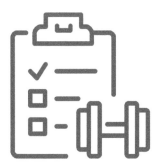

COPING WITH DOWNTIME

From time to time, we need to step away from running. The most common reasons are when we've sustained an injury or have come down with an illness. Whatever the reason, it's almost always frustrating. The best thing to do is pre-program some downtime into your training calendar to allow your body time to recover from a tough race or training block and help prevent some of those unwanted breaks that tend to pop up from overtraining. Allow a two- to three-week period after each season to relax.

I am not a huge believer in cross-training during an injury cycle, as I feel like the energy you expend on the bike or in the pool can take away from the energy needed to heal from whatever ailment has derailed your training. With that being said, I do think light cross-training can be beneficial for maintaining good hormonal balance, and it's encouraged by most coaches and sport science researchers.

Off time from running can offer an opportunity to develop some new and positive habits, like mixing up your workouts at the gym or incorporating yoga into your weekly routine. When athletes start missing practices due to sickness, I tell them to be somewhat productive with their

EMOTIONAL CHECK-IN

Here are a few questions to ask yourself when you're going through a difficult time and may need to do an emotional check-in. These questions are designed to establish positive thoughts. Learn how to give yourself a good pep talk and you won't need a coach! You can be your own best cheerleader—it just takes a little practice.

1. What's the best way to care for and comfort yourself? When life gets tough and you feel like you've failed or are hurting, how do you comfort and be true to yourself?

2. Did you make a dumb mistake? Accept that you're human and move on when things don't go exactly right. Use the mistake as a reminder to be in the moment and be mindful.

3. How have you helped someone else in the past few days? What do you do for your community? (Whenever I have a hard day and things don't go as planned, or I'm feeling overwhelmed with work and responsibilities, I reflect on how much I contribute back to my community, my daughter's elementary school, and my family. I take a hard look at how I positively influence other people's lives, and this usually gets me out of my funk and rips me from my pity party.)

4. Have you had a major setback? Will things be fine in ten minutes? Ten hours? Ten days? Boil things down to their simplest terms. Take it one step at a time and focus on what's important first, then progress from there.

5. How bad is it, really? Was it just a poor performance? If so, why did it happen? Chances are (like, I bet $100), you had a complicated few days before a bad race or workout. Not sleeping? Sleep deprivation is usually a major reason for a poor performance. Even eating poorly can lead to terrible thoughts and anxiety. Get yourself back in balance. Nurture yourself with good foods and plenty of rest.

time and stretch their muscles regularly. When an athlete has an injury that takes more than a few weeks to recover from, I sit them down and help them strategize the best, safest way to come back, without re-injuring themselves. Once the injury has fully healed and they feel good enough to begin training again, I tell them to go ahead and take one or two more days off to allow their health to really set in.

The reality is, being injured can be depressing, and some people in your life may not totally understand why. You're not getting in your normal physical activity each day, which means all of those feel-good endorphins have stopped flowing. Maybe you're even gaining a little weight. You know it's not forever, but it's normal to feel bad and be less positive than usual. Just remember that you're not alone and you don't have to suffer through it. If and when this happens, make sure you reach out to those in your support circle—friends and family members outside of the running clique you're a part of. It might be hard for the nonrunners to understand what you're going through, but you need them more than ever during this sensitive time.

Use this time to gain some perspective, too. Know that as runners, we push our bodies so hard and so frequently that setbacks are bound to crop up. Try to think of your "off" time as an opportunity to recover, refresh, and then hit the reset button for a new start.

We are often (almost always!) our own harshest critics. And when you're competitive by nature, it's even more notable—all the more reason we need to learn how to recognize and nurture self-compassion. I'm not talking about self-pity or becoming immersed in your own problems at the expense of neglecting others. Nor is it self-indulgence, when you choose to excessively gratify your own desires without considering what's good for you or others.

And it's not self-esteem, either. They may seem similar, but self-esteem really focuses on a person's self-worth and value in the world, while self-compassion is caring for yourself. If someone is hurting, upset, or suffering, you immediately want to console them and not walk on by. Well, you should feel the same way about consoling yourself.

PRACTICE GRATITUDE

Kaizen is a Japanese concept that extols the merits of constant improvement. However, that improvement—and our sense of accomplishment—doesn't have to come from a timer or a finish line. Improvement comes from building who we are as a whole and unique person. Success and, inevitably, our happiness are much richer than a single event, victory, setback, or achievement.

People may fall in different places on the positivity scale, but we all have the privilege of changing our thoughts and quick judgments. The power to reframe the direction of our thinking has everything to do with our level of happiness and self-worth. The happier we are, the more we'll continue to pursue the best of ourselves in running and in life. What a great cycle to put ourselves in!

In running, business, or tending a household, resiliency and gratitude are the most common attributes found in long-term success stories. Resiliency is useful whether we reach a big goal or fall short of it. We mostly think of resiliency as the ability to bounce back after challenges and crises hit, but it can be equally important after reaching a big goal. For example, some runners may feel empty or purposeless after they finally qualify for and run the historic Boston Marathon. Being able to find yourself after tackling a big life goal is just as necessary as moving on after you fall short.

Kaizen also encourages us to pursue higher goals. However, as I mentioned before, those goals don't always have to be about chasing a personal best as an athlete—it could also entail racing in a city that has been on your bucket list. After all, running through the city is the best way to experience it!

HEALTHY MIND-SET TIPS

Be thankful: Gratitude is the most powerful of all virtues. Being able to identify people, places, things, and practices that you're thankful for is a wonderful practice. Instead of focusing your attention on problems and challenges, you are identifying solutions, beauty, and joy in your life. Practicing gratitude releases serotonin, dopamine, and oxytocin (neurotransmitters that make us feel good). Here's how to direct or create thoughts that serve you better.

Rethink tough emotions: Journaling your emotions to work toward a more compassionate understanding of them. Reread what you wrote and underline a sentence or two that offer a constructive point of view.

Don't be disappointed by your disappointment: Feeling this way does not mean you are a failure—it means you care about what you are trying to accomplish. Give yourself credit for being invested in the process and continuing to show up and pursue it. Think about (and be grateful for!) the persistence of Thomas Edison, who said, "I have not failed 999 times. I have simply found 999 ways how not to create a light bulb." He sat back down and tried again, so get back in your running shoes and keep striving.

Take frustration in stride: It's okay to have a bit of a short fuse, but then cut yourself some slack. You had different expectations, but you can choose to replace the frustration with flexibility. Think of yourself as a cartoon character, red-faced and all, stepping out of a puddle of frustration and doing yoga next to it. Limber, calm, go through the stretches. Now that you're standing on more solid ground, think about your next move.

Ease sadness with gratitude: Sadness or melancholy is a heavy emotion to carry around. It's also a step in grieving, whether you've lost a loved one or an ideal race or a moment that slipped by. Or maybe it's reoccurring and you just can't seem to catch your breath. Any which way, the emotion is due to losing something you love or have been devoted to. Identify your loss, but be grateful to have loved or pursued someone/something that inspired you to feel so much. Then do something for yourself to spark a little joy. Maybe you'll find it outdoors, in nature. Or maybe you could bring nature into you, with fresh flowers or a new plant. Reflect on your gratitude list or write a whole new one. Contrary to popular belief, your mind cannot multitask, so if you're focused on gratitude, then sadness and frustration recede into the background.

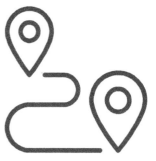

SECRETS OF A HAPPY RUNNER

I have a good friend who lives just south of Mammoth Lakes, in the little town of Crowley Lake. Nancy Fiddler is an avid runner and a two-time Olympian in Nordic skiing. She's also in her 60s. Nancy continues to run and hike in summer and is on her skis every day during winter. I recently chatted with her about her seasonal periods of training. She doesn't run in the winter months, which allows her body to recover from all the pounding and punishment the sport produces, but then once spring comes around, she'll start back up with the activity she hasn't done in months, and it feels like a fresh beginning. Nancy doesn't race anymore, but she still makes a point to be at every weekly track practice during the summer so she can compete with the younger men on our team!

Living a simple lifestyle in a small town in the mountains is right up Nancy's alley. She's a five-minute drive to our local public track, which is surrounded by some of the most beautiful terrain in the world. Her husband, Claude, reaps the benefits of this location, too. He was a fixture in Yosemite Valley in the 1970s and '80s, setting some of the most challenging rock-climbing routes that people still enjoy today. Talk about an active couple!

Nancy really excels at understanding the true value of recovery, especially as she gets older. She will take a day or two off if she feels like a body part is getting a little sore. Nancy has always been good at listening closely to her body. She has enough confidence in her athletic ability to know that taking a day or two off here and there will not amount to a significant decline in fitness—and in fact, it will only make her stronger in the end.

I would say that Nancy is a prime example of an athlete who has adapted well to aging. Sure, she knows that her best times are behind her, yet she still manages to stay in fantastic shape all year-round. Whether she's on snow in the winter or on dirt trails and track during the summer, Nancy manages to train intensely while balancing it out with rest and recovery. This is how she has set her priorities:

- Attend weekly Tuesday morning practice every week she's home.
- Do core work two to three times per week, for 15 minutes, without fail.
- First thing in the morning, drink a big glass of water, then eat a couple pieces of toast with a cup of coffee.
- Go to bed early and wake up early every day.
- If she doesn't feel like going out for a run, she'll put on her running clothes and just go for a walk. She usually ends up running after five or ten minutes, which results in (happily) logging a few easy miles.

Why does Nancy continue to run? Because she loves feeling strong and fit, and it motivates her in all aspects of her life.

Put anxiety in its place: I'll call this excitement, because the two emotions feel a bit the same internally, but anxiety feels too clinical while excitement gives me power. This is the art of reshaping your thoughts and emotions. If you're anxious for a race (or a promotion, presentation, etc.), try to see your life beyond that moment. Sometimes we obsess over a single, fleeting moment in our lives as if it's all we have going for us. Envision yourself after the event, enjoying time with friends or family, walking the dog, doing dishes to your favorite music, or reading another good book on the couch. More often than not, after some time goes by, we realize that whatever was making us anxious was actually preparing us for much better things to come.

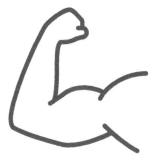

MIND-BODY WELLNESS TOOLS

In our never-ending search for the fountain of youth, we've found many ways to create and maintain a healthy relationship with our bodies, minds, and nervous system.

Introducing new stimuli and challenges promotes growth. Below is a list of a few activities that can challenge your mind and body to continue to grow. They're all designed to meld the mind, body, and spirit into one harmonious being and will benefit you physically and emotionally at any age.

YOGA

As we all know, yoga improves flexibility, but there's a wide range of health benefits that come with following the practice as well, especially if performed regularly with an instructor you know and love. Honestly, better flexibility is merely a wonderful bonus for us runners.

Consistently practicing yoga can bring dramatic health benefits over time, such as:

1. Providing strength for achieving optimal posture, which in turn keeps you "tall" throughout the day and leads to smooth and rhythmic breathing.

2. Building strength in your bones and muscles reduces the risk of muscle strains and fractures.

3. Increasing blood flow. Twisting movements, in particular, provide a wringing effect of our tissues and internal organs, pushing out stagnated blood and replacing it with fresh, nutrient-rich blood.

4. Draining your lymphatic system leads to improved immunity.

5. Cultivating a happier and healthier lifestyle. You're working on being more present, learning to ground yourself in stressful situations, and hanging around like-minded people.

Yoga—especially restorative asanas, guided relaxation, and pranayama—can also calm your nervous system and help you achieve deeper sleep. Practicing yoga slows down our thought loops of frustration that cause stress, creating a more peaceful mind. And never underestimate the power of a good instructor. They should be able to guide you and relax you in a way that few others can, so you truly get the most out of every session.

MINDFULNESS MEDITATION

Simply put, this is the practice of being present, controlling your thoughts, and redirecting them for the benefit of your health and those around you. There are a few different types of meditation out there, each providing you with a variety of ways to guide your thoughts in a healthy manner. Many of these practices are derived from Buddhist traditions and have been adopted by Western society. The base of all these different practices is the concept of mindfulness. The definition, according to Jon Kabat-Zinn, Ph.D., a molecular biologist and meditation teacher, is "an awareness that arises through paying attention, on purpose, in the present moment, non-judgmentally."

It can be difficult to commit to a meditation class if you've never tried one before. That's what I love about Headspace. It's a downloadable app for your smart phone that can guide you through many types of meditation and calming exercises. It's easy to follow and completely nonintimidating. If you're curious about meditation, it's a great way to jump in with both feet in the privacy of your own comfortable surroundings.

Practicing mindfulness meditation on a regular basis is often used to manage depression and anxiety as well as ease chronic pain. The combination of a calmer mind and a healthy diet has been shown to reduce inflammation in the body, which builds up over time. Having a calm mind leads to better food (and life!) choices, in general.

QIGONG OR TAI CHI

I like to think of tai chi (pronounced tie-CHEE) as yoga and meditation rolled into one. It's a low-impact and relaxing activity that consists of a series of 19 movements and one pose. It can have restorative effects on your body and mind. You may have seen a group of senior citizens practicing these moves in a local park, which is further proof that it's good for you at any age. But you don't have to be old to reap the benefits.

According to the Mayo Clinic, tai chi is an ancient Chinese tradition that was originally developed for self-defense and is now practiced today as a graceful form of physical and emotional exercise. The benefits of tai chi are similar to that of yoga and meditation:

» Decrease in stress, depression, and anxiety

» Improved flexibility

» Improved muscle strength

» Improved mood and energy

Qigong is another mind- and body-calming activity that integrates posture, movement, breathing technique, self-massage, sound, and focused intent, according to the National Qigong Association.

TIME IN NATURE

Do not underestimate the value of connecting with nature and the great outdoors. That's honestly one of the benefits, I think, of being a runner. We spend so much time outside, logging miles, breathing fresh air, and surrounding ourselves with nature. But we could all use a little more time outside, no matter where you live or how often you run, if you ask me. I'm fortunate to live in the mountains, surrounded by trees and lakes and hills, but I'll be the first to admit that I don't hike nearly as much as I should.

Having my daughter has made me realize that it's important to step outside, explore a new trail, and share that experience with someone. I guess if I lived near the beach, I'd have sand between my toes as I write this book.

Believe it or not, there are big health benefits to stepping out and connecting with nature, too.

» Improves short-term memory

» Reduces stress

» Can increase vitamin D levels

» Improves sleep

» Increases happiness

» Improves vision

» Inspires creativity

» Increases spirituality

Use nature walks and exploration as a time to unplug from the daily grind. We all spend way too much time in front of screens throughout the day, answering texts on our smart watches, responding to emails on our desktops, and scrolling through our social media on our smartphones. And with each passing year, our amount of screen—and sitting—time increases. Stepping onto a trail and leaving your phone in the car is a nice reprieve to give your eyes a rest and your mind a breather.

JOURNALING

In my wife Deena's book, *Let Your Mind Run*, she talks about the importance of writing a gratitude list each day and how journaling can be another way to lead a more mindful existence.

Here's an excerpt on gratitude from her book: "When we're grateful, we're immersed in goodness, and our brain is, too. Gratitude activates regions in the brain associated with the neurotransmitter dopamine, one of the body's feel-good chemicals. It's also associated with greater resiliency, optimism, motivation, better sleep, low anxiety, fewer aches and pains, and overall better health."

Self-expression can be so important, too. Writing, drawing, painting, ceramics,

sculpting, and creating music are all types of self-expression that can fulfill our desire to be creative. We all have unique traits we can share with others. I encourage you to pursue your creative side and don't be afraid to both challenge and express yourself. By doing so, you open yourself up to the opportunity to connect with others in a meaningful way.

I challenge you to create a list of five new ways in which you can express yourself to your family, friends, or community. Being a little more open and vulnerable with those you love, letting them see a side of you that you've never shared before, is good practice for any potentially difficult experience you may face together in the years to come.

STRIDE ON

I hope if there's one thing you've learned from this book, it's this: Running into and through your twilight years is more than just possible—it's preferred. And with the right tools and resources, anyone (yes, you!) can do it gracefully and graciously.

Ever since I was a young coach in Mammoth Lakes, I've always admired those "old guys" still kicking it at the local track every week. I personally try to lead a lifestyle and follow a training and nutrition regimen that will allow me to become one myself someday. I'm so happy to be able to share that knowledge with you, too. We've touched on a lot of topics—how to achieve optimal cadence, exercises to reduce inflammation and increase flexibility, foods that keep your ticker strong, ways to boost your emotional and mental health through running, and more—all in an effort to keep you running for years to come.

Can you visualize yourself in 10 years? Are you running strong and powerfully, racing in the local Turkey Trot or a fun 5K? If you can see it, you can be it. There's the person you're aspiring to be. Keep your head up and run in that direction. Lift others up around you as well. We'll need more support every mile and every year.

Continue to learn. Read, ask questions, discuss fun and exciting topics with others. Be social, share your knowledge of how to be healthy with others, spread the word about the benefits of yoga, tai chi, vitamin D, and resistance training! My wife and I have a motto: If you have it, share it. You have money, donate. You have time, volunteer. You have experience, offer it. Contribute, give back. It will make you a better, stronger, happier person.

Plan destination races with friends and family. I was just at the New York City Marathon (I go every year for work and to spectate) and I took my daughter out to dinner the night before the race. We sat next to a big family from San Francisco, and they were all there supporting "Grandpa" who was "carbo-loading" before hitting the streets of New York the next morning. It was going to be his 15th marathon, and he wanted to share the experience with his whole family. YES! This, my friends, is what running through the ages is all about. Share the experience, inspire others with your positive actions, and know that your steps on the track and off can help make this great world go 'round.

Despite what your younger self might think, you don't need to run fast to feel good about yourself or make a difference. I happen to be married to a fast marathoner, but when people meet her, they don't usually comment on her speed. Instead, they say, "You've inspired me to be a better person, to keep lacing up my shoes, and to keep logging the miles in pursuit of my goals." The elites don't inspire us by their fast times—they inspire us by their tenacity, their grit, their dedication to pursuing excellence and mastering their craft. So just give it your best in running and in life. Aim to be a little better at something today than you were yesterday. I hope this book helps you get there.

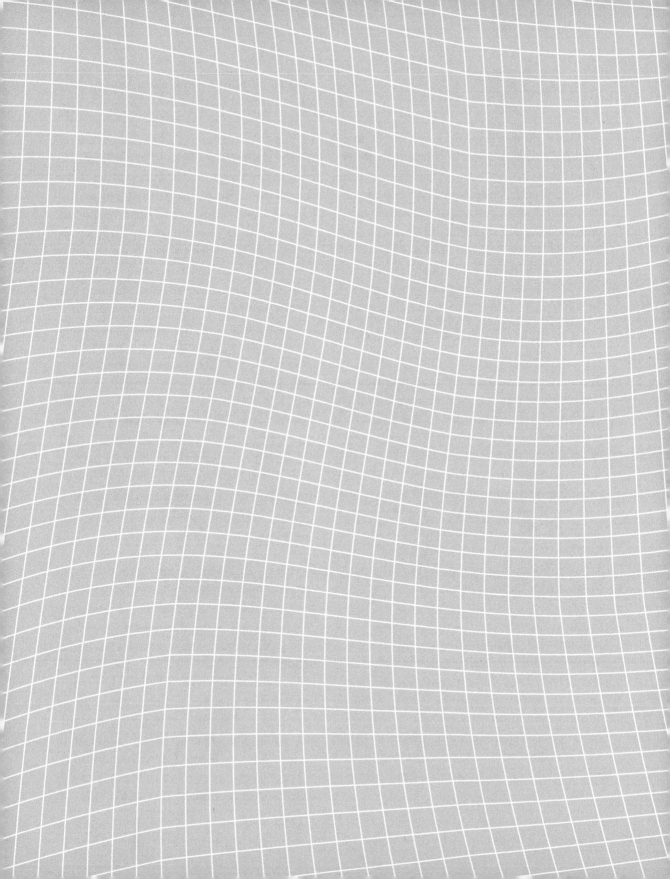

GLOSSARY

Achilles Tendonitis An overuse injury of the Achilles tendon, a bundle of strong tissue that connects the calf muscles to the heel bone (calcaneus) and produces power at push-off when running. Discomfort or a mild ache is usually felt in the back of the leg, just above the heel bone. The main cause of this injury is repetitive trauma—in the form of tearing—due to excessive stress in training. To prevent, try to avoid increasing training intensity and/or volume too quickly.

Bipedalism Derived from the Latin words *bi* (two) and *ped* (foot), this is essentially the act of walking upright on two limbs as a primary form of movement. Humans are bipeds. Most mammals use four legs to run with, so they are known as quadrupeds. Walking and running on two legs gives us a lot of advantages, including a greater field of vision (since our heads are lifted) while we move, plus the ability to wade in high water, access tree fruit, and carry weapons for fighting or hunting.

High Hamstring Tendinopathy A common condition in runners, this occurs when chronic inflammation develops at the origin of the three hamstring muscles, or the spot at the base of the pelvis (ischial tuberosity). Otherwise known as . . . wait for it . . . a pain in the rear! People afflicted with this condition often describe the pain as a vague, dull ache that usually limits stride length. Symptoms are more pronounced when running uphill.

IT Band Syndrome (ITBS) This unfortunately common overuse injury affects the connective tissue that runs down the outer thigh, from the pelvis to just below the knee. A sharp pain—usually strong enough to stop you in your tracks—is usually felt on the lateral aspect of the knee. Inflammation occurs when the stress on the IT band itself becomes overwhelming and the fibrous tissue starts to fray, one fiber at a time. My biggest (and best) piece of advice for runners with ITBS is to strengthen their adductors (groin muscles) to alleviate lateral knee pain.

Kinesiology The scientific study of the many physiological, biomechanical, and psychological aspects of human movement. It's such a vast and complex subject that colleges and universities tend to offer various types of specialized degrees in kinesiology.

Patellar Tendonitis This is a common running injury that affects the tendon that connects the kneecap (patella) to the tibia or shinbone. The main causes are overuse (repetitive forces with foot strike) or tight quadriceps (thigh) muscles, performing an excessive amount of downhill running and/or ramping up training volume too quickly. Discomfort and pain are felt just below the kneecap. If left untreated, it could lead to severe (i.e., career-ending) damage of the tendon, so this needs to be addressed immediately after detection.

Physiology A discipline of biology that delves into the routine and organized functions of organisms and their various structures. Human physiology, for example, looks at all of the complex systems of the human body that work together to make life possible, such as organ systems, anatomy, cells, biological compounds, and the interactions of all of the aforementioned. Colleges and universities offer various levels of degrees and disciplines within the broader study of physiology.

Plantar Fasciitis In my opinion, this is the worst possible running injury out there, because it can linger for years in some cases. Plantar fasciitis is the inflammation of the fibrous tissue on the bottom of the foot that is responsible for making the toes flex. When present, pain and discomfort is usually felt at the base of the heel and is usually most severe in the first few steps out of bed in the morning. This injury has the tendency to get "better" after warming up, but it will, unfortunately, revert to being sore once a training run is completed.

Runner's Knee (Patellofemoral Pain Syndrome) This is the most common knee injury among runners, hence its name. Pain and inflammation are caused by a misaligned kneecap that continuously irritates the femoral groove. Tight quadriceps can cause misalignment of the kneecap to occur, which leads to rubbing against the femur. Pavement pounding, or the repetitive stress of running, in general, can cause pain and inflammation in the kneecap region, especially when wearing worn-out shoes that don't provide ample cushioning or support.

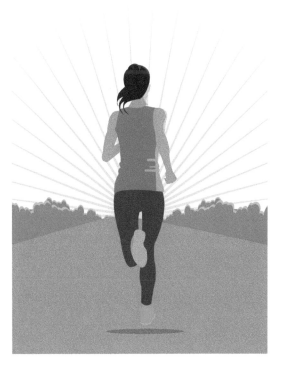

RESOURCES

I encourage you to delve a little deeper into some of the resources that I consulted when writing this book. I've written a sentence or two on each about the information I gleaned.

MOVIES

Spirit of the Marathon, 2007, directed by Jon Dunham. Distributed by Image Entertainment (US). This movie documents the journey of several athletes as they tackle the training leading up to the 2005 Chicago Marathon. Many marathoners watch this movie during their own marathon buildups as a source of inspiration.

PODCASTS

C Tolle Run with Carrie Tollefson.
www.ctollerun.com

Carrie Tollefson is a 2004 Olympian at 5,000M and a good friend of ours who interviews running's top athletes for her weekly podcast, *C Tolle Run.* Her interviews of professional runners give her listeners valuable insight, tricks, and tips. Carrie is also a TV commentator for many running events throughout the world.

The Morning Shakeout with Mario Fraioli.
www.themorningshakeout.com

Mario is a friend of mine who interviews a variety of athletes and coaches from around the world. My favorite podcast of his is with legendary Welsh marathoner Steve Jones. Mario is a host that knows how to get the best and most useful information out of his guests.

WEBSITES

United States of America Track and Field organization. www.usatf.org

Based in Indianapolis, USA Track & Field (USATF) is the national governing body for track and field, long-distance running, and race walking in the United States. This website is a great resource for all ages, from master's athletes to boys and girls looking to find national championships in all disciplines related to track and field.

Road Runners Club of America.
www.rrca.org

Based out of Arlington, Virginia, the Road Runners Club of America has been the industry leader in advocating for runners of all ages and abilities. Their organization compiles a wealth of resources for individual runners as well as running clubs in America. Use this website to find a coach or training group in your area today.

Podium Runner. *www.podiumrunner.com*
Newsletter via email.

Jonathan Beverly is the former editor in chief at *Running Times* Magazine. His website offers the latest research on training, running shoe reviews, and special commentary from top professional runners. Jonathan's newsletter gets delivered right to your email inbox about once a week.

REFERENCES

CHAPTER 1

American Heart Association. https://www.heart.org/en/. A good resource for helpful healthy guidelines for all Americans.

World Health Organization. "10 Facts on ageing and health." Accessed November 9, 2019. https://www.who.int/features/factfiles/ageing/en/.

Collins, Lois M. "Ageism is costing this country billions. Here's how." *Deseret News.* Accessed November 21, 2019. https://www.deseret.com/indepth/2019/9/24/20880106/elderly-media-portrayal-ageism-us-economy-aarp. An eye-popping account of how the elderly in the US are being treated and why.

Olympicchannel.com. "Ageism is the new sexism, says trailblazer for women's rights in sport." Accessed November 11, 2019. https://www.olympicchannel.com/en/stories/news/detail/50-years-later-kathrine-switzer-is-fighting-a-new-discrimination/.

Roizen, Michael F., M.D. and Mehmet C. Oz, M.D. 2007. *You: Staying Young, The Owner's Manual for Extending Your Warranty.* New York: Free Press. This is an extremely comprehensive book for all who are aging. And it's funny, too!

Trimble, Tyghe. "Why Japan is the most running-obsessed culture in the world" *Men's Journal.* Accessed November 11, 2019. https://www.mensjournal.com/entertainment/why-japan-is-the-most-running-obsessed-culture-in-the-world-w209376/ article, based on the book by Adharanand Finn, *The Way of the Runner: A Journey into the Fabled World of Japanese Running.*

McDougall, Christopher. 2009. *Born to Run: A Hidden Tribe, Superathletes, and the Greatest Race the World Has Never Seen.* New York: Random House, Inc.

CHAPTER TWO

Lovett, Richard A. "Mastering running as you age." Accessed October 17, 2019. https://www.runnersworld.com/advanced/a20852502/mastering-running-as-you-age-0/. This site provides a lot of real-life "how to" advice for runners of all levels.

Knight, Kathryn. "Arm swinging saves energy." Accessed October 19, 2019 *Journal of Experimental Biology.* The Company of Biologists Ltd. 2014. https://jeb.biologists.org/content/217/14/2431.1

Kastor, Andrew. 2017. *Running Your First Marathon: The Complete 20-Week Marathon Training Plan.* Emeryville, CA: Rockridge Press.

Wharton, Jim, and Phil Wharton. 1996. *The Whartons' Stretch Book*. New York: Three Rivers Press. I have given out this book and have reordered it time and time again for clients to reap the performance benefits of Active Isolated Stretching. It highlights the specific stretches and moves to maximize performance and time efficiency.

CHAPTER THREE

Bozeman Wellness Center. "Shoulder pass through—shoulder mobility." Accessed October 23, 2019. http://www.bozemanwellnesscenter.com/shoulder-pass-through-shoulder-mobility/.

The Matrix (1999) Warner Bros. Village Roadshow Pictures.

CHAPTER FOUR

Bjarnadottir, Adda. "How much caffeine in a cup of coffee? A Detailed Guide." Accessed November 5, 2019. https://www.healthline.com/nutrition/how-much-caffeine-in-coffee.

Oshin, Mayo. "The Blue Zones diet secrets from people who live up to 100." Accessed November 21, 2019. https://mayooshin.com/blue-zones-diet/.

Runner's World. "Calculate your calorie needs." Accessed November 21, 2019. https://www.runnersworld.com/uk/health/weight-loss/a766022/calculate-your-calorie-needs/. This site is instrumental in calculating your calorie needs as a runner.

CHAPTER FIVE

BAA.org. This site is useful for finding eligible courses for qualification into the country's oldest and most prestigious marathon, as well as the qualifying-time standards. https://www.baa.org/2019-boston-marathon-qualifier-acceptances.

Kastor, Deena. 2018. *Let Your Mind Run: A Memoir of Thinking My Way to Victory*. New York: Three Rivers Press. Deena went to the ends of the earth to produce a fantastic read on her personal journey of achieving peak performance through positive thought processes.

Neff, Kristin. "Self-compassion." Accessed November 7, 2019. https://self-compassion.org/the-three-elements-of-self-compassion-2/. Knowing how to love yourself is the beginning of living your best life.

Mayo Clinic. "Tai chi: A gentle way to fight stress." Accessed November 8, 2019. https://www.mayoclinic.org/healthy-life-style/stress-management/in-depth/tai-chi/art-20045184.

National Qigong Association. "What is Qigong?" Accessed November 8, 2019. https://www.nqa.org/what-is-qigong-.

Fetters, K Aleisha. "How to achieve that elusive runner's high." Accessed November 6, 2019. https://www.runnersworld.com/training/a20851505/how-to-achieve-a-runners-high/.

INDEX

ABOUT THE AUTHOR

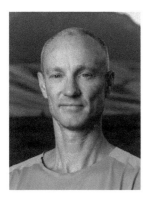

Andrew Kastor started his running career in the early 1990s at the age of 14, when he competed in cross-county, track, and road racing while attending Fountain Valley High School in Southern California.

He then went on to pursue a degree in Exercise Physiology from Adams State University in Alamosa, Colorado. While in college, Andrew's commitment to the sport of running continued to grow, and he competed in cross-country and track, specializing in middle-distance events.

Post-graduation, Andrew moved to Mammoth Lakes, California, where he created and coached a nonprofit running club called the High Sierra Striders. He's now the head coach for the Mammoth Track Club.

Andrew currently resides in Mammoth Lakes with his wife, Deena (Olympic Marathon bronze medalist and American record holder in the marathon), and their daughter, Piper Bloom.

PROFESSIONAL HIGHLIGHTS

» Coaching director for the L.A. Marathon and Los Angeles Road Runners (2012–2015)

» Coached Shadrack Biwott to fifth place in the 2016 NYC Marathon and fourth in the 2017 Boston Marathon

» Has coached 15 Olympic trials qualifiers

» Authored the book *Running Your First Marathon: The Complete 20-Week Marathon Training Plan* (2018)

» New York Road Runners online coach (2008–2010)

» Head coach for Mammoth Track Club (2012–current)

» High altitude training consultant for International Athletes

» Marathon coach for Saudi Arabian Olympic Committee— Rio 2016

» Contributor to various national print publications, including *Runner's World, Running Times, Shape, Fitness, Health, Women's Health,* **and** *New York Runner*

» Continues to work professionally with runners of all abilities— from Olympians to Boston qualifiers to first-timers